Low-Fat Living
for Real People

LOW-FAT LIVING
for REAL PEOPLE

The Fat-Free Chocolate-Covered
Creme-Filled Mini-Cakes Diet
and Other Confusions of Low-Fat Eating
❧ EXPLAINED ❧

BY
LINDA LEVY
AND
FRANCINE GRABOWSKI, M.S., R.D.
REGISTERED DIETITIAN, NUTRITION COUNSELING CENTER,
HAHNEMANN UNIVERSITY HOSPITAL, PHILADELPHIA

Drawings by LINDA LEVY

Lake Isle Press, Inc. / New York

Book design: Christopher Kalb
Cover design: Karen Katz

September 1994
10 9 8 7 6 5 4

Contents

Contents

Acknowledgments

Like a major motion picture, this book has been "years in the making," and there are many people who have helped us. For their generous giving of time to read manuscripts: Deborah Lowden Donahue, M.A., R.D.; Parichehri S. Sami, M.S., R.D., C.D.E.; Susan Brozena, M.D.; and our "lay person," Dorothy Brecht, who read and listened and commented and was ever-helpful. We are most grateful to the ALS team, particularly Marlene Ciehoski and Sharon Hulihan, who are models for excellent health care and nurturing, and to Patricia Joynt, M.P.S., C.N.S.D, R.D., for her leadership, problem-solving skills and professional guidance, as well as to the ARA managers at Hahnemann University Hospital, who enthusiastically support our goals. We thank Dennis Helms, who advised us not only as a lawyer but as a friend, and Denny Siegel, professionally trained in the culinary arts, who gave us many useful suggestions.

There are others who lent their ears and their help, too: Joan Frieder, who always knew what to say – and when; Shelly Margolis and Laurel Kreeger, who gave up Wednesdays; Tony De Santis, who gave his love, energy, good nature, and music; Marie Cascone, who provided us with all sorts of esoteric information; Jo Brozoski, who inspired us to write a book that people could actually read; and Princeton Public Library, whose reference staff was invaluable. We thank our parents, Julius and Julia; John and Jane; and our children, Jeff, Valerie, Deborah, and Tim; Theresa, Michael, Jennifer, and Leigh Golding, for thinking this whole project was more than just a good idea. We thank Karen Katz for her cover design; Chris Kalb for his book design; and Victoria Mathews for her wonderfully sensitive attention to editing matters. And we thank Lake Isle Press and Hiroko Kiiffner, whose good humor, good sense, and good grace have made this project possible.

Foreword(s)

Take a family whose favorite dinner was fried chicken and buttery mashed potatoes, whose idea of a great bedtime snack was ice cream (preferably vanilla fudge) with potato chips on the side, who thought the good life had something to do with thin-crust pizza with extra cheese.

In other words, take our family.

My husband and I have three children, the oldest two of whom were already away at college when the New Regime went into effect and we changed our eating habits. (The youngest refers to himself as "a foot soldier in the war against fat.") We had a reason for making the change.

It was a memorable day in March 1987 when the doctor said that my husband, who had experienced some discomfort in his chest, would have to have his heart "looked at." My husband pretty much wears his heart on his sleeve, but apparently that wasn't good enough – nor were the so-called "noninvasive" procedures (elaborate x-rays, stress tests, et cetera) that followed.

We couldn't imagine that anything could be wrong. Years ago this man had learned to confine his cigarette smoking, never very heavy in the first place, to the golf course. (If he were a golf pro, that wouldn't have been much help, but he isn't.) Although his job certainly falls into the sedentary category, he is very active otherwise, has never been over-weight, and has never had a cholesterol reading in the bell-ringing range.

No, we couldn't imagine that anything might be wrong. But we were wrong. Cardiac catheterization, a hospital procedure that allows doctors to see the heart from the inside, revealed that there was some blockage in one of the main heart vessels, and so angioplasty was performed. (This is just like catheterization, except that a tiny balloon is inserted into a blocked vessel and is inflated and pushed through the vessel to clear away the fatty deposits.)

We learned from the cardiologist that many individuals in the United

States over the age of forty have blocked arteries, which can lead to a heart attack. Sometimes you don't know how these things are going until it's too late. We felt lucky to have had a warning.

We learned, too, that studies are showing that the problem begins early in life. Autopsies on the bodies of once-vigorous young men in their late teens have revealed fatty deposits already forming in the heart vessels, a terrifying thought.

The good news is that changes in the way we eat can actually improve our chances of living a long and healthy life. Sounded good to us, and gave new meaning to the phrase, "The way to a man's heart is through his stomach."

Having cooked for a long time, I had my special recipes. In fact, when I heard that a friend was putting her favorite recipes on the computer, I resisted the urge to ask if she would henceforth be doing her cooking in the family room, where the computer is located. And I realized that my cookbooks and I had a system of our own; my favorite recipes were spattered with a number of their key ingredients, which served to wrinkle the pages so that I could open right to a particular recipe whenever I wanted to. At least as efficient as a computer.

I must say modestly that I am a good cook. Still, having established certain patterns over a quarter of a century, it was not easy to make many of the changes that were necessary. In fact, as I look back on it, I was in what I have come to call a "culinary depression" for about four months, months when I experimented with new recipes in an effort to make healthy dishes. I spent hours in the supermarket reading labels so that I could locate acceptable (from the standpoint of fat content) products. And I was afraid that the food I cooked would be terrible. Well, the food I cooked *was* terrible. I followed recipes of the cook-your-way-to-a-healthier-heart type that said things like "Slice an eggplant. Place it under the broiler until golden. Enjoy!" (Okay, okay, I made this up, but you get the idea. "Enjoy" we didn't.)

As I gradually became accustomed to cooking edible yet healthy foods, I met Francine Grabowski, a registered dietitian who helped us to "eat smart" – and collaborated with me on this book. We found that we share a basic philosophy, one that is summed up by the old saying: "Give a man a fish, you feed him for a day. Teach a man to fish, you feed him for a lifetime." Aside from our mutual concern about the woman who appears nowhere in this saying, probably because she is at home cooking the fish in question, we realized that books giving rules are the equivalent of giving a fish. This book is a fishing lesson.

It took a long time, but the happy day came when I realized that I could cook food that was not only healthy and edible, but also absolutely delicious and very, very easy to prepare. Together, my husband and I learned to read labels and to ask appropriate questions when ordering in restaurants. With three other couples, we formed a gourmet club for healthy eating, meeting at each others' houses for potluck suppers that didn't involve cream sauces and thick cheese toppings. They, like us, were beginning to try to eat in a way that didn't scream "1950!" The eight of us became a support group, called ourselves "Ate is Enough," and had shirts made with the logo we designed: a cheeseburger with a line through it. The group continues to this day.

And so to *Low-Fat Living for Real People.* There are currently on the market all kinds of books about all kinds of problems for all kinds of diets. These diets deal with sugar, with salt/sodium, and so on. (Your doctor may have recommendations concerning your own particular diet.) But just about everyone seems to be dealing with the issue of lowering fat, and that's what this book is all about.

"Ate is Enough" support group

▶

It is for you, whether you have had a problem already (fear is the great motivator), or whether you can simply read the hand-writing on the wall. It will spare you a lot of what we went through in learning to adapt to a new lifestyle, and in learning to cook wonderful, quick-to-fix dishes. It will show you how to get your family on your side, how to eat out, but most important, how to live in this world. And I do mean live.

This is serious business, but it doesn't have to be depressing.

– Linda Levy

I'll never forget the 1994 Winter Olympics. A horrified television audience went behind the scenes to watch figure skater Tonya Harding frantically attempting to fix a broken skate lace as her name was announced. I was watching Tonya's coach.

It occurred to me then that a dietitian is a trainer/coach, setting up the right conditions for people to succeed, and cheering them on through countless days of practicing, stumbling, learning new skills. But there is a big difference: The training is not for a moment of glory at an Olympic event; it is for a lifetime.

For years I have coached people through life-saving nutrition changes, decreasing the risk of damage from heart disease, certain types of cancer, and diabetes. Those who have won their personal battles would agree that this is worth more than any gold medal.

More often than not, nutrition counseling occurs at a time of crisis. (Whoever said, "Necessity is the mother of invention" must have been a dietitian.) During my years at Deborah Hospital, a leading heart hospital in New Jersey, I became keenly aware of the fear, disbelief, and over-whelming stress caused by the crisis of disease, not only for the patients themselves, but also for their families. I saw the enormous need for "coaching," for knowing the best nutritional techniques to help in their particular condition, for tapping the great reservoirs of courage we all have, and for providing actual, realistic strategies in the way of lifestyle changes designed to ensure success.

The "realistic strategies" have to take into account that people are busy, that change is difficult, and that a set of rules takes away from the pleasure of eating. Real people worry that it takes a lot of time to plan new meals, or to experiment with lower-fat versions of their old stand-bys, much less learn a new recipe. And they worry that the food won't taste good.

Low-Fat Living for Real People shows that they don't have to worry. Small changes are the answer and can make a significant difference. Furthermore, with gentle, good-humored coaching, all changes become easier, more natural, and less painful. Not coincidentally, I hear clients say, "I feel so good! I have so much energy!"

There are those who say the available information is confusing, and if you are among them, you are not alone. There is confusion about even the most basic nutrition. To the dismay of dietitians everywhere, information about the good foods like vegetables, fruits, and starchy beans just can't compete with advertising budgets like those of McDonald's, Coca-Cola, and Kellogg's. Therefore, people often need help to find their way through the maze of nutrition misinformation. A registered dietitian, who has had years of special training, is uniquely qualified to provide this help.

There are also times when a dietitian works with a person who has given the time and energy to learning about low fat, who knows that nutrition is a critical step in managing serious medical problems, and who has created a joyful style of low-fat living. This is how it was when I met Linda. Truly a leader, inspiring families and friends, designing new recipes, taking every suggestion and making it better, her energy is contagious and inspirational.

Low-Fat Living for Real People is more than just "real information." It is also about staying healthy, being creative, and having fun.

– Francine Grabowski, M.S., R.D.

Chapter One

Leaving the Fat Behind

Getting the Facts Straight

First, a word from our sponsor:

Cholesterol

Yes, we, the food-buying public, are being sponsored by cholesterol. For years we have seen it everywhere, *everywhere*, particularly in its most popular form, "NO CHOLESTEROL."

Whoever thought that one up must still be laughing. Why? Because the words "no cholesterol" may be found on items that never in a million years would contain cholesterol anyway. Because *cholesterol is found only in animal products* (meats, fish, eggs, cheese and other dairy products).[1] So when potato chips brag that they don't contain any cholesterol, well, those wafer-thin slices of potato have been fried in vegetable oil, so there's no earthly reason for them to contain cholesterol in the first place.

No, oil may not be cholesterol but it sure is fat, F-A-T, and you can be darn certain you'll never see "NO FAT" on a package of good, old-fashioned potato chips that you've known and loved for years. But cholesterol is the buzz word, and manufacturers realize that we know a little something about it, but not too much, just enough to know we don't want it, so what the heck, they figure they'll point out that their product is cholesterol free.

This whole business is further complicated by the fact that it's all too easy to confuse cholesterol in your *diet* and cholesterol in your *blood* ("serum"), which are not the same thing. If your doctor has ever taken a look at your lab results and said, "We're going to have to do something about this cholesterol," that was serum cholesterol he or she was referring to. (Speaking of doctors, any dietary changes made for a medical condition will need a doctor's supervision. This book is not a substitute for professional care.)

Because there appears to be a powerful link between high serum (blood) cholesterol and heart disease, people are trying to lower choles-terol, and there is a great deal of information out there on how to do it: Eat plenty of fiber, raise the "good" cholesterol through exercise, and so on and on and on. Yes, there is information, much of it dry, some of it confusing, and not what you'd call eminently readable.

The fact of the matter is that serum cholesterol is partly under your control and partly inherited. Let's talk about one thing we *can* control: food.

♦   ♦   ♦   ♦

I t's natural to assume that limiting cholesterol-rich foods in your diet will lead, automatically and inevitably, to lower cholesterol in your blood, and will improve the health of your heart. Sad to say, you could fill many a grocery cart with cholesterol-free foods, but these same foods could still be very high in fat. In fact, according to Jane Brody of *The New York Times*, considered by more than a few people to be the patron saint of health and fitness, "Far more important than the cholesterol eaten are the total amounts and kinds of fat in the diet."[2] In other words, restricting fat is the thing to focus on when you want to eat more healthfully. Why? Because a low-fat diet has many health bene-fits, not the least of which is that it helps prevent clogged arteries, and may also decrease the risk of developing certain kinds of cancers. A nice bonus is that a diet low in fat will result in weight loss, which in itself will help your heart. Indeed, if you have not lost weight, chances are that your low-cholesterol diet is, nonetheless, high in fat. On the other hand, a diet low in fat will also be low in cholesterol. (Organ meats – brains, liver, kidneys – are the exception and should be avoided. They are low in fat but high in cholesterol.)

Okay, so we're getting the idea that cholesterol is not the only villain in all this. But how to proceed?

By reading labels.

CHAPTER **1**

Leaving
the Fat
Behind

*"Far more important than the cholesterol eaten are the total amounts and kinds of fat in the diet."
– Jane Brody*

•

A diet low in fat will also be low in cholesterol, unless you are eating a lot of organ meats – brains, liver, kidneys.

Getting Organized

Reading labels is definitely the first step in getting organized, because labels will guide you through the miles of supermarket aisles and help you decide what foods to buy (or not to buy). The labels look complicated, but don't despair. Do the best you can for the moment, and by the time you come to the chapter that explains just how to use these labels to select low-fat foods, you'll find that *Low-Fat Living for Real People* has given you the necessary background to do that. You will be able to sift through and interpret the label information, and make it work for you.

Label Reading

Granted that labels are destined never to make the best-seller list, and that they are boring, boring, boring, but there's no getting around it: that's where the information is to be found. Unfortunately, labels are not made for easy reading, and, for those of us growing more farsighted by the millisecond, it seems as though they are printed in letters the size of a pinhead inscription of the Lord's Prayer. It would be a whole lot easier if crackers, for instance, came in a laundry detergent-sized box that could accommodate labels with VERY LARGE PRINT.

But they don't. So even if it means putting on your reading glasses in order to see labels clearly, it makes sense to read them if you're trying to eat less fat. You'll soon be convinced to buy differently, since many of the old standbys will be out-of-bounds. Take the time to check out the products that you buy routinely, such as crackers, cereals, cookies, and so on, and you'll be amazed to see the fat lurking there. Simply because a food is light, crisp, and non-greasy, you might assume that it is low in fat. You could, we're sorry to say, be mistaken, because fat may be precisely the ingredient that is providing the crispness.

The fringe benefits of label reading are enormous. Because you'll feel less and less inclined to buy some of the items that you've been buying for years, you'll discover that there are long stretches of aisles in the supermarket you can avoid, thus dramatically cutting down on your shopping time. While the initial visits will take longer as you establish new buying habits, that won't last, and soon enough you'll be back on automatic pilot, mindlessly throwing groceries into the cart the way Mary Tyler Moore did every week at the beginning of one or another of her television shows while the titles ran. The only difference will be that you'll be throwing different things into the cart than you used to, and certainly different things than Mary Tyler Moore did.

The Pyramid

Remember the Four Food Groups (sounds like they might have had a hit single in the fifties)? They have been replaced by the Food Pyramid, introduced to Americans as a model for healthy eating, and useful also as a handy guide to foods that are low in fat. In fact, the Food Pyramid is the newest and best time-saver of them all.

Why a time-saver? Because it can help you decide quickly and easily which foods to buy. Then, as you stand in line at the check-out counter, pretending you're not looking at the tabloid headlines, you'll be confident that you've filled your cart with "all the right stuff."

You will save not only time but brain power if you simply fill your shopping cart with starches, fruits, and vegetables (all low in fat); the Food Pyramid honors all of these by placing them at or near the broad base. By contrast, put little in your cart in the way of fats, oils, and sweets, which you'll find perched in the tiny section at the top of the Pyramid.

As for the milk and meat level, the fat content is, unfortunately, not so clear-

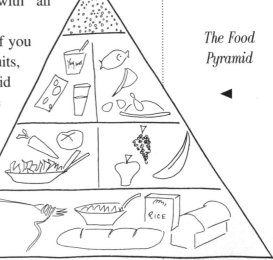

*The Food
Pyramid*

Leaving

the Fat

Behind

cut. For instance, you'll see beans with meats, since both are high in protein. But unlike meats, beans are low in fat and high in starch. They coexist happily with the other starches at the base of the Pyramid and can be eaten in the greatest quantities.

So how do we know what to do with meats and dairy products? Never fear. *Low-Fat Living for Real People* will help you a bit later in this book.

You'll see that the Pyramid specifies how many servings of a given category should be eaten in a day, but don't worry about exact amounts. Instead, think of the Pyramid recommendations as relative. Plan to eat, for example, more pasta than meat. If there is a Food Pyramid drawn on the box of your favorite cereal, consider cutting it out and putting it on the refrigerator as a handy reference (hint: wait until the box is empty before cutting).

The Wonderful World of Grocery Shopping

This is a very, very good time in the history of the Wonderful World of Grocery Shopping to be leaving the fat behind. You'll want to fill your shopping cart with foods that are pleasing in their taste and texture, foods whose colors are so appealing that they look wonderfully inviting on the plate. Variety is not only the spice of life, it is actually the basis for a healthy diet. Fortunately, it is a simple matter to increase the variety of foods you consume, now that supermarkets have grown to such a size that some of them deserve to have their own zip codes. They are stocked with all sorts of surprises.

Bell peppers, for instance, are now available in more than just traditional Christmas colors. Yellow, orange, and even deep purple ones can be found. Tropical and out-of-season fruits and vegetables are also commonplace these days. Besides the mushrooms that look like the little drawings in children's stories, there are others: shiitake (tiny parasols), huge Portobello (beach umbrellas), enoki (large toothpicks with tiny hats), to name a few.

Frozen vegetables have gone far beyond peas and carrots to include such items as asparagus, artichoke hearts, and snow peas. Ethnic foods are readily available – bean sprouts, water chestnuts, flour tortillas. Beans, both canned and dried, come in a wide variety: kidney, pinto, lentil, split pea (green and yellow), black-eyed pea, chickpea (alias garbanzo or ceci), Great Northern, navy, black, pink (rosetta), and even a bean called simply "small white bean."

We've come a long way from bread shelves stocked primarily with the soft white stuff that some people think of as "raw," others think of as "the bread that doesn't spoil," and still others think of as "the bread you can play with." Bakery sections now feature all sorts of freshly made loaves, from white to whole grain.

Other aisles offer fresh as well as dried pastas, all of which come in shapes and sizes to suit your every mood. Vinegars have gone beyond red, white, and apple cider, and are flavored with herbs and fruits. Mustards are made in all sorts of interesting varieties, so you don't have to choose between the old standbys, the brown one and the bright yellow one that you find at sports stadiums and that make you want to break into a chorus of "Take Me Out to the Ball Game." The new mustards have names like "coarse and sassy" and may be made with wine, dill, honey, or champagne.

Tomato products, formerly pretty much limited to ketchup and tomato paste and canned tomatoes, today include crushed plum tomatoes with basil, pasta sauces, and the increasingly popular salsa (which just means "sauce" in Spanish, but where's the fun in calling it that?). Yogurts can be found that are nonfat; some have fruit added, which may or may not be pre-mixed. One man we know was eating his first Dannon apricot yogurt, unaware that it required stirring, and was wondering why in the world it was called "apricot." "And then," he reported, "I hit gold!"

Leaving

the Fat

Behind

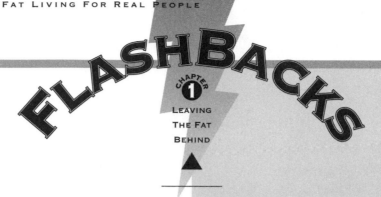

FLASHBACKS appear at the end of each chapter and are reminders of the key points in that chapter. (They should look familiar, and if they don't, you may want to go over the chapter again.) If you don't remember one other thing about *Low-Fat Living for Real People*, including who wrote it, please, please, PLEASE remember the **FLASHBACKS**.

☞   End all confusion about cholesterol; **choose low-fat or fat-free products.**

☞   **Eat plenty of starches, fruits, and vegetables.**

☞   **Be adventurous in the supermarket:**
Try a new fruit.
Try a new vegetable.

Chapter Two
Jack Sprat's Favorites

Jack

Sprat's

Favorites

J*ack Sprat could eat **low** fat,*
His wife could eat no lean.
And so betwixt them both, you see,
He outlived her by a long shot.

–Nursery Rhyme, updated

Best Bets: Starches

I t's fine to talk generally about food and recent advances in food, but what, you might well ask, are good choices? Which leads us neatly to the subject of STARCHES.

It may be, in an age when everyone talks about "complex carbohydrates," that when you think of starch, you think of laundry and ironing, but in fact starches are complex carbohydrates and this is as good a time as any to bring the word back into vogue.

There are people who already feel comfortable with starches, who naturally steer clear of fat-laden foods. They eat a vegetarian diet, lean toward organic produce, have an herb garden and a compost heap – and are not buying this book.

At the other extreme are people whose food choices are quite different, who believe that potato chips contain all the essential nutrients, who think that brown eggs are somehow healthier than white ones, who get their exercise by lying on the couch and watching workout videos, and who wish this whole thing about eating less fat would simply go away, the way that business about converting to the metric system did. (Although it didn't go away entirely. We'll be dealing with grams and milligrams on the food labels, and you can't get much more metric than that.)

Most likely you fall somewhere in between the two extremes, getting kind of anxious about this low-fat business, but not quite sure how to go about making what seem like earth-shattering changes in lifestyle. You will be delighted and relieved to see that many of the foods you recognize and already buy are actually good for you.

Chances are that these foods are starches, and what makes them "good" is that they are very low in fat or fat free, and are therefore low in guilt or guilt free as well. An extra added attraction is that starches may even help control weight. In fact, studies show that all calories are not created equal, and that extra calories taken in as starch are less likely to result in weight gain than are extra calories taken in as fat.[3] Life can be beautiful.

So what is it that makes starches (the edible parts of plants: wheat, corn, rye, barley, rice, potatoes) so attractive? In addition to their weight-control appeal, they contain fiber, vitamins, and minerals. By the way, you should know that all plants contain a tiny bit of naturally occurring fat, but this fat does not contribute to heart disease. On the other hand, some starches contain added fat, which makes them less desirable.

HOW DO YOU KNOW IF THERE IS **ADDED FAT** IN BREAD, FOR EXAMPLE?

You'll know if the Ingredient List on the package includes butter, vegetable shortening, or oils. Notice the difference between these two bread labels:

HEARTY-STYLE WHOLE WHEAT: Enriched wheat flour, whole wheat flour, *hydrogenated vegetable oil (may contain cottonseed or soy oil)*, salt, flavoring.

HEALTHY BAKERY: Whole wheat, oats, rye, rice, corn, buckwheat, millet, water, wheat bran, salt.

◆ ◆ ◆ ◆

Because starches are about to become your new best friend, let's take a look at them from the standpoint of stocking your kitchen cabinet. After all, if your shelves are loaded with fatty foods, that's what you'll eat. On the other hand, if those are starches in the cupboard, you'll be well on your way to better eating before you've even opened your mouth.

Think again of the Pyramid introduced in chapter one. You'll remember that it can help you make healthy choices – "all the right stuff" – quickly and easily. What follows is a pyramid of one particular type of food: starches. Again, the bottom of the pyramid contains foods that may be eaten in the greatest quantity, in this case starches that contain no added fat. That is, you will not find any fat in the list of ingredients. At the top portion of the pyramid, starches do contain some fat. As a single food, eaten in a reasonable quantity, they present no problem. Still, if you are trying to limit the amount of fat you are eating, everything counts, so while you're at it, you might as well go with the no-fat-added starches in the bottom of the Pyramid of Starches.

The Pyramid of Starches*

L o w - F a t
CRACKERS
(melba, saltine, gra-
ham, J.J. Flats, Nabisco
Harvest Crisps and
Triscuits, Venus bran wafers)

RICE (brown, white, wild);
GRAINS (barley, couscous, bulgar
wheat, air-popped popcorn); **BEANS**
(dried, canned): kidney, lima, lentil, split
pea, navy, chickpea, etc.; **PASTA** (formerly
"spaghetti"); **POTATOES** (white, sweet);
BREADS; **BAGELS** (fat free); nonfat **CRACKERS**
(matzo, Finn Crisp, Wasa, Ry-Vita, Nabisco Fat-Free
Saltines, Health Valley Fat-Free Crackers); nonfat
CEREALS (hot, including oatmeal, grits, cream of wheat,
oat bran; cold, including Kellogg's Corn Flakes, All-Bran,
Grape-Nuts, Cheerios, puffed cereals, shredded wheat); **PRET-
ZELS** (fresh-baked soft pretzels; Snyder's of Hanover Sourdough;
other fat-free pretzels); Happy Heart No-Oil Corn Chips; Guiltless
Gourmet No Oil Tortilla Chips; Near East Rice Pilaf, Lentil Pilaf, Spanish
Rice; **STARCHY VEGETABLES** (corn, peas, acorn and butternut squashes)

*There are other foods made with starches–for instance, angel food cake, Entenmann's fat-free bakery products, fat-free Hostess Light Twinkies, fat-free SnackWell's products–that have not been included in the Pyramid of Starches because they do not offer the nutritional benefits of starches found here. Even though these foods contain flour (starch), they also contain a lot of sugar, and while sugar is "fat free," so to speak, and provides quick energy, it is without the health benefits of starches. In addition, eating sugary foods reduces the likelihood that you'll eat "good" foods – fruits, vegetables, and the kinds of starches that appear in the Pyramid of Starches. To find out more about sugar in the foods you eat, check the Endnote.[4]

Note that this is not an exhaustive list, and that, where brand names are included, they are intended as suggestions, not endorsements. Similarly, brand names that do not appear may indeed suit the above criteria, but space – and shape – prevent listing them all. Not to mention the fact that new products are coming into supermarkets every day. *Careful label reading, particularly the Ingredient List, will tell you specifically what products to buy and will guide you in choosing starches that contain no added fat.*

Obviously, the more you eat of a food that contains even a small amount of fat, the more fat you get. Because of fat content, serving size becomes a key issue in the upper section of the Pyramid of Starches.

Own Personal Serving Size (OPSS)

When manufacturers give information about fat, calories, and so on in their products, they use "serving size" as the reference point. This is fine now that most food labels are based on a serving of food that a person might actually eat, which gets away from the old problem of foods being divided into unnaturally small servings so that the per-serving information would look more appealing to the consumer. Still, *the serving size on the label may not bear any resemblance to the amount you, personally, eat.* Check the label to see what is considered the serving size, and then match it with your Own Personal Serving Size (OPSS). The next time you pour yourself a bowl of breakfast cereal, for instance, measure what you normally eat. If it's two cups, fine. That means the serving size of your cereal is two cups. But what if the box says the serving size is half a cup?

The serving size on the label may not bear any resemblance to the amount you, personally, eat.

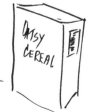

*The label
law has
defined "low
fat" as 3
grams or
less per
serving.*

Well, now you are eating *four times* the serving size on the label.

Let's suppose the label says there are 3 grams of fat per serving. The label will often say that, too, because the label law has defined "low fat" as 3 grams or less per serving.[5]

You have to do a little math to see how much fat you are actually getting in your two cups of cereal. Since your OPSS is four times that which appears on the box, you have to multiply the fat by four to find out that you have – all together now – 12 grams of fat per serving. A little high, wouldn't you say? You might want to switch to a lower-fat brand of cereal rather than cut your OPSS down to half a cup and find that you are starving by ten o'clock in the morning.

> **If "grams" are unfamiliar, don't worry.**
> A gram is simply a unit of weight, about that of a straight pin, and 28 grams are equivalent to something you are familiar with: one ounce.

So we see that it's not enough just to go with foods that say they contain no more than 3 grams of fat per serving, because your serving size might be considerably bigger than the one listed on the label, in which case those grams of fat are adding up faster than video game points. To keep this from happening, you'll want to stick to the starches that contain no added fat.

One fine day (in our dreams) starches will edge out meats as the centerpiece of the American diet. What this will mean is that, if you serve dinner on the kind of sectioned plate once used for "Blue Plate Specials," the largest section will contain not meat, but starches, perhaps pasta or potatoes or a rice dish, and the meat (or chicken or fish) will go into a smaller section. In fact, you'll be able to answer the infamous question "What's for dinner?" without automatically mentioning first the meat, or chicken, or fish.

Beans, the All-Star Starch

On some level, we have known for a long time that beans are good for us. There was even a childhood rhyme about beans being good for the heart, a rhyme that we were not allowed to say in front of grown-ups. (If you'd like a refresher lesson, turn to the Endnote[6]

**Starchy
Beans**
*black-eyed peas
cannellini
chickpeas
fava
kidney
lentils
lima
navy
pink
pinto
split peas
white beans
whole peas*

for the prime time version.) The undesirable side effect, namely, flatulence, or gas, will be less of a problem as your system becomes accustomed to eating beans.[7] A few drops of a product called "Beano" (available in pharmacies), when added to the first forkful of beans that you eat, may also help.

Beans really are good for us. Why? Fiber, fiber, fiber. STARCHY BEANS (dried or canned)[8] are low in fat, too. In fact, you'll see them right there in the big, lower section of the Pyramid of Starches (see page 26).

Beans come in a wide variety of colors, shapes and sizes, and can be used in many dishes. Canned beans are the easiest to use. Drain and rinse them well (they'll be less salty) and throw them into just about any soup – vegetable, chicken, whatever – or toss them with your salad. Or you can open the can of beans a day ahead and put the rinsed, drained beans in a bowl with some fat-free bottled dressing, then let the whole thing marinate in the refrigerator until you toss that salad. Or add the beans to frozen, mixed vegetables (thawed but uncooked), and marinate together (see recipe for Marinated Beans and Vegetables, page 167).

Dried beans are fine, too, but they require presoaking plus a couple of hours or so to cook. You can soak them overnight in cold water, or you can boil them for two minutes and then let them sit (covered) for one hour. In any case, discard the soaking water and add fresh before cooking according to package directions.

Be aware that you might possibly find a little rock or two in the package along with the dried beans. These have to be removed, because, unlike beans, they will not soften no matter how long they are cooked. When we say that beans contain minerals, this isn't what we have in mind.

Beans offer a pleasant change of pace. One day when you find yourself in the supermarket idly wondering when they'll invent a new meat, try beans. Beans are in the mainstream now; you'll even see them on the

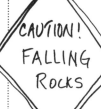

CAUTION!
FALLING
ROCKS

Jack

Sprat's

Favorites

Fruits
apples
apricots
bananas
blackberries
blueberries
cantaloupe
cherries
dates
figs
grapefruit
grapes
honeydew
melon
mandarin
orange
sections
mangos
nectarines
oranges
papayas
peaches
pears
persimmons
pineapples
plums
prunes
raisins
raspberries
strawberries
tangerines
watermelon

menu in nonvegetarian restaurants. Recipes are all over the place, too. You'll find them on the bags and cans in which the beans are sold, as well as in cookbooks and newspapers and magazines – and in the back of this book, for that matter. Just make sure that your recipe follows the low-fat recipe rules on page 132. You may be surprised by how much you like beans.

Best Bets: Fruits and Vegetables

There are other complex carbohydrates that contain virtually no fat but do contain plenty of vitamins and minerals, the old standbys, as well as other amazing goodies, some as yet unidentified. As a package – that is, as food – they are essential to a healthy heart, and may indeed protect it from disease.[9] These complex carbohydrates are the ever-popular FRUITS AND VEGETABLES. When we studied nutrition ("Health") with Miss Miller back in sixth grade (she wore her hair in a bun, didn't believe in lipstick, and made sure her long, gray cardigan sweater was buttoned up to her neck), fruits and vegetables were one of the basic food groups, and they're still around. Unlike some other food groups we could mention, they have never fallen out of favor. Remember Carmen Miranda with her hat loaded with fruit? Turns out it was a low-fat hat.

While fruits and vegetables retain their celebrity status – we should be eating five servings a day – not everyone actually eats them. *Moby Dick* remains a great book, but does everybody read it?

Consider fruit. Close to *half the population* is apparently too busy to eat any fruit at all.[10] Sobering, when you consider that not much in the way of preparation time is needed to peel a banana, let alone simply bite into an apple (as Adam found out, to his dismay). They are the ultimate easy-access fruits.

As for vegetables, preparation is required, which isn't exactly enticing. They have to be peeled, sliced, diced, chopped, minced, or grated.

Food processors can help, unless left untouched in the kitchen cabinet. If used, they have to be dismantled, washed, and then reassembled, all of which can be off-putting for people who don't get much more high tech than that little gadget that removes apple cores. But there is another way to get your vegetables, one which you may find more–ahem–palatable. Think "salad."

Salad

Eating salad is, of course, a great way to get your vegetable quotient for the day, and there is a tool-free approach to its preparation, one that doesn't even involve a knife or cutting board. In the supermarket you can buy everything you need, already cut up and ready to go. You'll find tiny little carrots, peeled and washed; shredded cabbage; cute little pieces of broccoli, ditto cauliflower; sliced mushrooms; bite-sized cherry tomatoes. You may even find washed, packaged lettuce leaves.

Or you can spin your own with a salad spinner, a wildly useful tool and a boon to people who used to let their lettuce dry on towels spread all over the kitchen – and dining room, too, if lots of company was coming.

As long as you are spinning lettuce, remember that iceberg lettuce is almost entirely devoid of nutrients. You have only to remember the Titanic to know that icebergs don't have what you'd call an enviable reputation, so you might want to think about selecting another, darker green (and therefore better for you) lettuce, such as romaine. Romaine will keep for several days in the refrigerator if it has been washed, spun, and bagged in plastic. You could also use spinach, bibb lettuce, or another leafy green, or even a combination of these. You might even add those marinated beans mentioned earlier, throw the whole thing together, and make one spectacular, prize-winning salad.

CHAPTER 2

Jack

Sprat's

Favorites

Vegetables
artichokes
asparagus
beans
broccoli
brussels
sprouts
cabbage
carrots
cauliflower
celery
cucumbers
eggplant
greens:
beet
chard
collard
dandelion
kale
mustard
turnip
leeks
mushrooms
okra
spinach
sprouts
squash
zucchini

Jack

Sprat's

Favorites

Other Time-Saving Approaches

Frozen vegetables are another option, and require only opening a box or tearing open a bag (Scissors? Knife? Teeth?), making it easier than ever to eat vegetables with all their heart-protecting qualities.

Last choice (mushy, bland, salty) but better than no vegetables at all are the canned versions hanging around on the supermarket shelf. (It's seven o'clock. Do you know where your can opener is?) They can be heated, dumped into soup, or used as weights in an aerobics class.

But what if you don't like vegetables, have never liked vegetables, have absolutely no interest in eating vegetables? For your heart's sake, consider that they have come a long way from the days when they were a soggy, beige side dish. As we've just seen, without even being cooked, they can be put in salads. Lightly cooked and tossed with chicken or fish, they add flavor, color, and texture. Fully cooked and puréed, they can be used as a sauce. Overcooked, they can be thrown out.

But beware of prepared (and incredibly expensive) frozen and packaged vegetables, because in the preparation process – that is, while they're adding sauces and gravies and cheeses and so on – they're adding fat at the same time. Read labels carefully. All too often there is more fat in these things than you can imagine, and considerably more than the 3 grams per serving that is the current standard for "low fat." Not to mention the fact that your OPSS (Own Personal Serving Size) may well be bigger than the one indicated on the package. Although it seems easier to use these products, the trade-off is simply unacceptable.

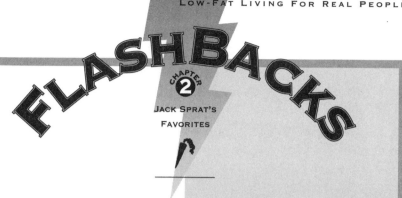

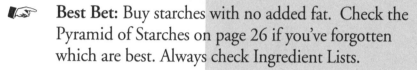

Best Bet: Buy starches with no added fat. Check the Pyramid of Starches on page 26 if you've forgotten which are best. Always check Ingredient Lists.

In the running: Buy starches with a little added fat. Make sure there are no more than 3 grams of fat per serving. More than that is too much.

Try BEANS! Versatile, delicious, and easy to use, they are the All-Star Starch.

Create a modern "Blue Plate Special" that features grains, beans, or pasta in the largest section of the plate.

Pay close attention to your OPSS (Own Personal Serving Size). The bigger your OPSS, the more fat you are getting.

Other Best Bets: Buy (and eat) fruits and vegetables. Count your blessings – salad counts as a vegetable!

Chapter Three
Protein Reconsidered

Center Stage No More: Meat and Poultry

Meat and poultry have customarily occupied a privileged place on the dinner table, the main event at the main meal of the day. When we remember the Sunday roasts of our childhood, we conjure up a scene that Norman Rockwell would have been crazy about. We remember a heavily laden dinner table with bowls of mashed potatoes, boats of gravy, baskets of buttered biscuits. We remember quantity, going back for seconds and maybe even thirds. We remember good food, good times, good feelings, with an occasional squabble over who would get the end cut.

Back when a "roast" referred only to food, not to a bunch of individuals making wisecracks about some honoree, people loved eating it. But why put it in the past tense? There are a lot of families out there who still love it, who know that the best way to make sure the kids come home for dinner is to announce that a roast will be served. Even older, married kids can often be lured back this way. Beans and rice just don't hold the same fascination.

The taste of a roast, like anything else, is acquired, and the fact is that you've simply gotten used to eating it, lots of it, maybe. Possibly you have weekly barbecues where you roast something enormous on a spit in your backyard.

Or it may be that you have cut down on your meat eating. After all, these aren't the first words you've read on the subject of reducing fat in your diet, and you might well have gotten wind of the fact that meat is where a lot of the fat is. So let's say you're eating less meat, and that you're making do with a life-sized, full-color cardboard cutout of a medium-rare roast beef in the middle of the table in lieu of the real thing.

When people are eating less meat, they're often eating chicken instead, low in fat yet comfortably familiar. You're probably already doing that, and you can feel confident that you are moving in the right direction. (This assumes, by the way, that you are not eating chicken *wings*, which are, unlike other parts of chicken, high in fat.)

If you're on a real poultry binge, chances are good that you are eating so much chicken you have come to the point where you say things like "If I see another piece of chicken, I'll grow feathers." That's a sure sign that you have fallen headlong into the dreaded chicken rut, and are tired of building your meals around chicken. The best way to climb out of the chicken rut, without going back to mashed potatoes, gravy, buttered biscuits, and roast beef, is to introduce yourself to some starches, fruits, and vegetables that you might have overlooked in the supermarket. The "embarrassingly simple recipes" at the back of this book will help you.

We must be clear on this: We are not saying you should give up meat. Or chicken, for that matter. We are saying you might want to take another look at them – how often you eat them, and how much you eat at one time.

*Introduce
yourself to
some
starches,
fruits, and
vegetables.*

◄

A Little Goes a Long Way

Cutting down on the amount of meat and poultry you eat will, at the same time, reduce the amount of fat you consume, including Mr. Big of the fat world, SATURATED. It all comes down to the fact that *cutting down on your serving size is the most important of all dietary changes.* Yet people balk at doing this. Maybe they have old myths ringing in their ears, something about needing lots and lots of protein. But in fact you need to eat only small amounts of meat or poultry, because you don't need much protein each day.[11]

News *Flash*:

Your protein does not need to come from an animal or a fowl. It might come from beans, and it might come from whole grains and vegetables, too. Studies show that there tends to be less heart disease among people who eat vegetarian diets.[12] (There are different types of vegetari-

*Cutting
down on
your
serving size
is the most
important
of all
dietary
changes.*

Protein
Reconsidered

*The serving
size for
meat and
poultry is
3 ounces,
something
like a deck
of playing
cards.*

an diets, the strictest of which does not include anything that comes from animals. Keep in mind that a great many vegetarian recipes include animal by-products like eggs, cream, butter, and cheese, which makes them very high in fat. You can bet that these are not the kinds of recipes that were used in the studies just mentioned.)

We aren't suggesting that you become a vegetarian, only that you be aware that non-animal protein offers two advantages: ❶ You don't need to think about the serving size of chicken or beef or whatever; and ❷ you don't need to worry about fat. Take heart. Literally. You can do it.

Let's get back to serving size, because the fact is that most of us are used to eating meat or poultry every day. We've discussed serving size earlier (OPSS – Own Personal Serving Size), but it warrants more discussion here.

If you've ever been to a steak house, you've been introduced to outlandish portions that have absolutely nothing to do with what we're talking about here. A restaurant that serves meals whose centerpiece is 16 or more ounces of cow flesh really should be located near a heart hospital. Besides, a steak like this has to be served on an incredibly large plate – let's face it, a platter. Shouldn't you be able to fit your food onto a normal-sized dinner plate? If you find yourself eating from serving platters, you might want to rethink portion size.

Yessiree, a 16-ounce serving is outlandish, but it may be even more outlandish than you realize. The recommended serving size for meat and poultry is – you'd better be lying down for this – *3 ounces, something like a deck of playing cards.* No one is proposing that you share that 16-ounce steak with three friends (and even at that, you'd get more than 3 ounces), but the idea is to begin to cut down on serving size, which will cut down on fat, including saturated fat. Then, too, as you cut down on the amount of meat and poultry you eat, you will naturally eat more starches, vegetables, and fruits, which is the whole idea.

Also, as you cut down on these serving sizes, you'll be cutting down on cholesterol, since (we've said it before and we'll say it again) a diet low in saturated fat will also be low in cholesterol, unless you are eating a lot of organ meats.

When you cook your own meat, you may have heard that you should "allow for shrinkage," which is to say that the meat weighs more before it's cooked than after. That's true, but you can't buy a slab of meat the size of a Kleenex box and expect the cooked weight to be appropriate. To put it in perspective, if you buy a pound of lean ground beef, by the time you allow for shrinkage during cooking (25 percent), that pound of beef will make four heart-healthy, low-fat living hamburgers of about 3 ounces each.

That's LEAN Meat We're Talking About

If you're eating meat, what to buy? It's not which animal you eat, but what part of the animal. You want lean, not fatty. This goes for poultry, too. (By the way, most of the fat in chicken and turkey is housed neatly in the skin, so by dispensing with it, you are that much ahead. If you look underneath the skin, you'll also find a few unappealing little hunks of pale yellow fat, which should be removed before cooking the chicken.)

Up to this point in our discussion, we have talked about "low fat." But now we're talking about meat and poultry, and The Powers That Be instead use the terms "Extra Lean" and "Lean." Extra Lean has half the fat and saturated fat of Lean, and you don't have to bother going to butcher school, because you'll know that the meat or poultry is acceptable *provided you eat only 3 ounces.*

Buy "Extra Lean" or "Lean" meat.

Even if your meat department isn't using Extra Lean and Lean stickers, you can still get nutrition information, since the label law requires that it be readily available. However, that information might be anywhere – on the meat, on the counter, posted on the wall – or it might be scribbled on sheets of paper that are stuck underneath a cash register someplace, in which case you'll have to ring the bell and ask someone for the information you need.[13]

As for lunch meats, they often say "97% fat free." Sounds good, but this is very, very misleading, making you think the product is low in fat even if it isn't. Sometimes the manufacturers add a lot of water during processing.

Protein
Reconsidered

If they would take out the water (fat chance!) from a lunch meat that calls itself "97% fat free" and then show you the fat content, you'd see that the lunch meat may be as much as 50 percent fat, not 97 percent fat free at all. A good choice? We don't think so!

The fact is that certain lunch meats share only the vaguest family history with cows and pigs and chickens, which makes you wonder why they are called "meats" in the first place. They come packaged in perfect squares and circles and have names like "bologna" and "olive loaf." When was the last time you took your child to a petting zoo to see an olive loaf? Don't buy lunch meats and assume you are buying meat.

Now we'll tell you how to be certain you aren't paying for lunch meat pumped full of water.

Since water has no calories, you can believe that you're getting meat, not water, *if there are more than 60 calories in a 2-ounce serving of "97% fat free" lunch meat.*

Best Bet: Fish

All fish are appropriate for a heart-healthy diet.

Fish is a different, well, a different kettle of fish. It contains protein, all right, but fat is not an issue, even if you've heard some fish referred to as fatty. (Besides, there's very little saturated fat in any fish.) There are people who don't eat salmon and mackerel, for example, because they are fatty fish, but the truth is, all fish are appropriate for a heart-healthy diet. In fact, eating fish may very well be the easiest way to reduce the risk of heart disease.[14] Only if a fish is deep fried or otherwise cooked in a lot of fat is it the kind of "fatty" you'll want to avoid.

Naturally, if you eat a variety of fish, you'll get a a variety of benefits. You don't have to eat large amounts of fish, either. Just two meals a week, with a serving size of 3 ounces at each meal, will do the trick, an amount that will be, by now, a familiar quantity.

As for shellfish, which is very low in fat,[15] suffice it to say that it has an undeserved reputation for raising serum cholesterol. Enjoy it occasionally; there is no reason to avoid it, unless, of course, you are keeping kosher.

The recommendation to eat fish more frequently is really nothing new. But maybe you harbor a lingering resentment because of all those Fridays when you had to eat fish. Or maybe you think it smells bad (comedian Elayne Boosler asks, "How do you know when herring has gone bad? Does it smell good?"), but we assure you, fresh fish doesn't have an unpleasant odor. Then, too, when you think "fish," maybe you immediately think "fresh fish," which makes you think of making yet another shopping trip, which in turn makes you throw your hands up in dismay and opt for a nap.

"How do you know when herring has gone bad? Does it smell good?"
– Elayne Boosler

That extra shopping trip has to do, of course, with the fact that fish spoils easily and you can't just keep it around, although if yours spoils overnight, your refrigerator may not be as cold as it should be. Fish will keep longer if you put the package in a bowl filled with ice cubes before putting it in the refrigerator.

So if you can't keep fresh fish on hand, how about frozen? There's no question that it loses a lot in the translation, which is to say the freezing process, but it is certainly better than no fish at all. Frozen fish sticks, however, bear about as much resemblance to fish as ginger ale does to champagne, so don't go eating frozen fish sticks and think you're eating fish. Maybe when you were a kid you drank ginger ale and pretended it was champagne, but you probably don't want to eat

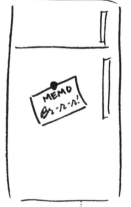

fish sticks and pretend they're fish. Besides, chances are that the breading has a lot of fat in it, the very thing you're trying to avoid.

Is your refrigerator cold enough?

But there is another alternative to fresh fish, and that is canned, yes, canned, convenient and easy to keep on hand. Needs no refrigeration, either. All right, so you're having a little trouble envisioning a long, flat can with a flounder inside. You may even be wondering why you never

Protein
Reconsidered

noticed it in the supermarket, an impressive can like that, somewhere near the tuna. We admit we've never seen canned flounder either, but to be perfectly honest, when we mentioned canned fish, we were thinking (besides tuna) of salmon. Some canned salmon has the extra added attraction of bones, and although you may doubt that anyone on this earth would want to pick out bones, we hasten to add that that's precisely the point: you don't pick out the bones. You shouldn't pick out the bones. They fall apart easily as you mash up the salmon and you'll never notice them, but they'll be there nevertheless, providing you with a nice source of calcium. A simple way to use salmon is by making a tuna salad using salmon instead (see recipe for Crunchy Tuna Salad, page 149), and if you want to feed a lot of people, you can buy salmon in a can big enough to be mistaken for soup. (If there's a center bone in that big can, we suggest you remove it, rather like you take out the center plug from a fresh pineapple that has been prepared by that exotic machine in the supermarket.)

Proceed With Caution: Cheese

People get their protein from meat, from poultry, from fish and shellfish. They also get their protein from dairy products in the form of milk, cottage cheese, yogurt, and cheese. Like all dairy products, cheese is an excellent source of calcium and protein but it is also an excellent source of fat.[16] Now, because we are a nation of cheese-lovers-who-are-trying-to-lower-their-fat-intake, cheese manufacturers have been playing around with low-fat, even no-fat, cheeses. They've had a few minor problems with the stuff, like getting it to melt. You might ask yourself just what it is you're dealing with. One woman put some leftover broccoli on a baked potato, topped it with fat-free cheese, and popped it into the microwave. When she took it out, the cheese was nowhere in sight. She found it later, when she'd finished eating the potato and broccoli. There it was, stuck fast to the plate.

As for the taste of the fat-free cheeses we've met–ohboyohboyohboy. You might as well send your taste buds on vacation. The cheeses are soapy, and some of them are so rubbery they actually bounce. (Don't ask how we happen to know this, but trust us. They bounce. Toys "Я" Us probably has a cheese aisle.) Still, even though the flavors and textures are nothing like the original, if you are of the persuasion that a day without cheese, not orange juice, is like a day without sunshine, then by all means go for it.

In fact, there are low-fat cheeses (no more than 3 grams of fat per ounce) that have been around for centuries, and, although they don't have the familiar ring of cheddar, mozzarella, and Swiss, they have the advantage of being untouched by modern technology. They have names like farmer's cheese, goat cheese, hoop cheese, and sapsago cheese; you might want to try them. You could also stay with old-fashioned cheese, the kind mother used to buy, and just use less of it. This is fine if you can convince yourself that 1/4 cup of grated Parmesan sprinkled over an entire casserole is enough. But if you can already picture yourself scraping off the entire cheese layer and putting it on your own plate, you'd do well to consider eliminating cheese from your day-to-day diet. This doesn't mean that you'll never have another pizza. It simply means that cheese moves away from the everyday and into the realm of "occasional treat."

Low-fat cheeses: *farmer's goat hoop sapsago*

Variety, Variety, Variety

Now that you know you can eat meat, poultry, fish and shell-fish, and cheese, the only thing left to do is to eat all of them. Over the course of a week, though, not all at once. And in 3-ounce servings, too. Remember the old adage, or something close to it: "Variety is the seasoning of existence."

Since different foods offer different benefits, plan a week's meals that include a variety of foods. Instead of serving chicken four or five nights out of seven, try the following pattern: chicken or turkey, two nights; fish or shellfish, two nights; vegetarian, two nights; one night, your choice. We chose leftover turkey, but you might choose beef or pork. Add a salad or hot vegetable and some fruit, and you have a complete, delicious, low-fat meal.

Monday
Shrimp with Tomatoes (see recipe, page 148) and rice

Tuesday
Grilled Turkey Breast (see recipe, page 142) and baked potato

Wednesday
"Mexican" Eggplant (see recipe, page 155)

Thursday
Rice, Pasta, and Spinach (see recipe, page 158)
with leftover Grilled Turkey Breast (see recipe, page 142)

Friday
Carefree Flounder (see recipe, page 145)
and Embarrassingly Simple Rice (see recipe, page 162)

Saturday
Bean and Pasta Soup (see recipe, page 171)

Sunday
All-Purpose Chicken (see recipe, page 139)
and Not Too Boring Potato-Onion Casserole
(see recipe, page 160)

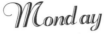

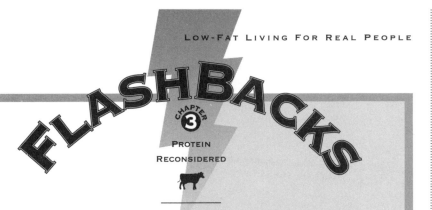

FLASHBACKS

CHAPTER
3

PROTEIN
RECONSIDERED

👉 Think "deck of cards," not "placemat," when it comes to the serving size of meat/poultry/fish.

👉 Choose "Extra Lean" and "Lean" meats.

👉 **If you eat lunch meats:**
Choose 97% fat-free lunch meats with at least 60 calories in a 2-ounce serving.

👉 **Take a break from chicken every night.**
Make fish, beans, or vegetables, rather than meat or poultry, center stage.

Chapter Four

Ms. Sprat's Favorites

Worst Bet: Saturated Fat

It isn't very hard to know what's what in the Fats World. Saturated fat is about the worst of the dietary offenders, the fat most closely associated with heart disease. A "killer fat," you might say. Doesn't sound all that great, does it? You've seen it rear its ugly little head in the meat/poultry/cheese combine, but it lurks menacingly in many other places as well: butter, cream, sour cream, cream cheese, ice cream, and other high-fat dairy products. The good stuff, in other words. This means that not only do we have to change the way we eat, we also have to change the rhymes we teach our kids: "I scream, you scream, we all scream for – nonfat frozen yogurt!"

On top of everything, there is another kind of fat, *trans* fat, that mimics the effect of saturated fats on the body. Growing more unpopular by the day, because it may well turn out to be even more harmful than saturated fat, it is found in (hard to spell much less pronounce) HYDROGENATED and PARTIALLY HYDROGENATED FAT.

*Saturated
fat and
trans fat
are the
gruesome
twosome.*

Worst Bet #2: Hydrogenated Fat

Ah, the wonders of modern science! A chemical process known as hydrogenation takes a poor, unsuspecting vegetable oil and changes it so that it becomes solid and spreadable (margarine, shortening), and lengthens the shelf life of the products it is found in. Good idea? No, bad idea, because the process results in the creation of both saturated fat and *trans* fat, the gruesome twosome when it comes to dangerous fats. Food labels won't help you spot *trans* fat, because, as of this writing, specific information on *trans* fat has no place on the label. But foods that contain hydrogenated or partially hydrogenated fat will say so on the Ingredient List.

And there are many such foods. Besides being found in lots and lots and lots of the packaged foods you buy (chips, crackers, cookies, and other commercially baked goods), hydrogenated fat is commonly found in margarine.

People are actually proud of the fact that they use margarine, brag about it to their friends, use it as a sign of how they've solved the problem of using too much fat, and therefore how they're protecting themselves against heart disease. They see margarine as a reasonable alternative to butter, but the truth is, thanks to the presence of hydrogenated fat, it isn't.[17] A far better alternative is jam or jelly, which contains no fat at all, but is, admittedly, not very useful for sautéing.

As far as fat content is concerned, *both butter and margarine are **all fat**.*[18] (Clarified butter is no better. The clarification process merely removes any "contaminants" and leaves pure, unadulterated fat.) What could be more fatty than the margarine that advertises itself as being "100% corn oil"? Even reduced-calorie, whipped margarines get all their calories from fat. It's just that the air that's whipped into them puffs them up so that there are fewer calories in a spoonful. But you must understand this: What calories there are come from fat. Remember, you don't need any saturated fat in your diet, and you certainly don't need a cheap imitation (hydrogenated and partially hydrogenated fat).

The newer margarines that contain no hydrogenated or partially hydrogenated fat – and no *trans* fat – are an obvious improvement (taste aside) over butter, but they are still all fat. They may even have fewer calories, but they are still all fat.

You don't need any saturated fat in your diet, and you certainly don't need a cheap imitation.

Ms.

Sprat's

Favorites

Better Bet: Monounsaturated Fat

Saturated fat is not the only fat; it is simply, as we've said, the worst offender. However, you must consider all kinds of fats, since TOTAL FAT is the issue here. Maybe we should coin a word and simply call all other fats "faturated." Let's examine them.

Apparently the best bet, from the point of view of heart health, is monounsaturated, of which olive oil and canola oil are prime examples. Those who live in Mediterranean countries have known the secret of monounsaturated fats for a long time, use olive oil in their cooking, and have a very low rate of heart disease.[19] Canola oil doesn't have the history of olive oil, but it may well have the promise.[20] If you are confused about what fat to use in cooking, you may want to go with these oils, but go easy: no more than one teaspoon added fat per serving. Nobody is recommending that you deep fry your pasta in monounsaturated oils.

SPEAKING OF OLIVE OIL, A QUICK DIGRESSION.

You might logically think that, if olive oil is a fat of choice, olives would be a good thing to eat. After all, where does olive oil come from? As a matter of fact, one of the writers of this book is a devoted olive fan. (We won't talk about the other.) But because olives are a fat, even though a particularly "good" fat (monounsaturated), you'll want to think of them as garnishes,[21] not main or side dishes, and use them accordingly, to enhance the taste and texture of other foods. The same is true for avocados and nuts, whose oils are also monounsaturated. (Chestnuts are an exception. Despite their name, they contain little fat.)

Ms.

Sprat's

Favorites

And Then There's . . . Polyunsaturated Fat

B esides monounsaturated fat, there is the famous polyunsaturated fat, very commonly used but losing its "good guy" status. Although it first appeared that polyunsaturates were innocuous even in large quantities, that now seems not to be the case.

What are some examples of polyunsaturated fat? Most of the oils that you use in daily food preparation are polyunsaturated. Some of these are: safflower, sunflower, corn, sesame, cottonseed, and soy. But you don't have to memorize long lists. You already know that olive and canola oils are monounsaturated – read "good." Fats of animal origin are saturated (as are tropical oils such as coconut, used less often in processing foods today than they used to be) – read "bad." Everything else is polyunsaturated.

WARNING:

In the products that you buy, polyunsaturated oils may be "hydrogenated" or "partially hydrogenated," so you can no longer consider them polyunsaturated. As we've said, as far as your body is concerned, they might as well be saturated. And it's worth repeating that, because they don't spoil, these disreputable fats are frequently found in margarine and in an enormous number of, indeed most, processed foods – crackers, cookies, and other commercially baked goods.

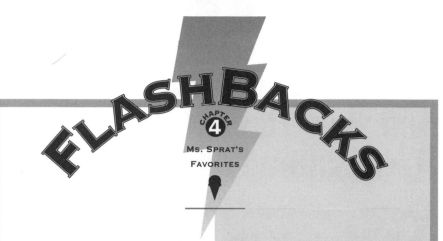

FLASHBACKS

CHAPTER
④
MS. SPRAT'S
FAVORITES

 Remember that saturated fat would be voted Least Admired by members of the Academy of Fats if there were such a thing. It is found in meat, in poultry, in cheese and other dairy products, and earns a definite "thumbs down."

 While you're at it, remember that both hydrogenated and partially hydrogenated fat are saturated fat copycats as far as the body is concerned. They are found in margarine, chips, cookies, crackers, and commercially baked goods, and also earn "thumbs down."

 Because of the hydrogenated fat in margarine, it is not a reasonable alternative to butter.

 Best Bets: Use monounsaturated fats, such as olive and canola oils.

 Because they are fats, avocados, nuts, and olives should be used only as garnishes.

Chapter Five
Sizing Up Fat

Sizing

Up

Fat

Understanding Quantities

Now that we know what kinds of fats are out there, let's talk about quantities, because we need to have some understanding of how much fat we are taking in, and how little we should be taking in, to help keep ourselves healthy.

FOOD WE MAKE: Normally when we cook our food, we measure in teaspoons, tablespoons, and cups:

1 tablespoon = 3 teaspoons
1/4 cup = 12 teaspoons (4 tablespoons)
1/2 cup = 24 teaspoons (8 tablespoons)

FOOD WE BUY: It's too bad that, when we shop for food, we are forced to think in the language of labels, that is, in GRAMS. We remind you that a gram is a very, very small unit of weight (there are 28 grams in an ounce), about that of a straight pin.

All cooking oils contain the same amount of fat, so don't be misled by special blends and the like. There are 5 grams of fat in a level teaspoon, whether oil or margarine or any other fat, unless it is one of the new, lower-fat versions. (Check labels. Nucoa Smart Beat spread lists 2 grams of fat per serving and no hydrogenated or partially hydrogenated fat, clearly the wave of the future.)

What follows is an easy-to-use conversion chart, showing how much fat (in grams) is found in common household measures:

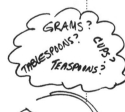

1 teaspoon oil = 5 grams
1 tablespoon oil = 15 grams
1/4 cup oil = 60 grams
1/2 cup oil = 120 grams
1 cup oil = 240 grams

Measuring in Grams, Courtesy of "The King"

You may or may not be happy to hear that Elvis Presley has come back from the dead (assuming you believe he's dead) to help us understand how to think in both kinds of measures, that is, teaspoons/tablespoons/cups on the one hand, and GRAMS on the other.

When we think of Elvis, we think of his hit song "Are You Lonesome Tonight?", which asks the musical question, "Is your heart filled with pain?" It's an excellent question indeed when you consider that Elvis reportedly had a fondness for red-eye gravy, which is almost entirely bacon grease. In fact, the drippings from one pound of cooked bacon (just to keep measurements simple), mixed with a little black coffee, makes enough red-eye gravy to pour over biscuits and serve four. Hazardously. (Hey, kids! Don't try this at home!)

We'll give Elvis's mother, Gladys, one thing: her recipe was undoubtedly embarrassingly simple. But if she had measured the drippings when she cooked that pound of old-fashioned, fatty bacon, she would have found there was just over a cupful, or 260 grams of fat from the whole pound of bacon, which means that one serving has *sixty-five grams of fat* (260 divided by 4). M-m-m-m BAD.

We bid a fond farewell to the ignorance is bliss era of the fifties and return to the present, when we are (or should be) concerned about the amount of fat we take in each day.

"ARE YOU FAMISHED TONIGHT?"

(To the tune of "Are You Lonesome Tonight?")

Are you famished tonight?

Are you famished tonight?

Are you sorry you can't eat much fat?

Does your memory stray

To your porterhouse days

When your steak was the size of a mat?

Does your vegetable platter

Seem overly bland?

Do your beans, rice, and pasta

Seem overly planned?

Is your heart filled with pain?

(Not if you're eating grain!)

Tell me, dear, are you famished tonight?

Sizing

Up

Fat

Spreading the Fat Around: A Daily Diary

Why worry about teaspoons, tablespoons, cups, or the 65 grams of fat in red-eye gravy? Because we're leading up to the idea that there's a limit to how much fat is appropriate to take in each day – on your bread, on your salad, in your cooking. The Big Picture.

In order to better understand the notion of quantity, we need to look again at margarine, a very commonly used, yet much misunderstood, form of fat.

How much margarine might you use in a normal day? It makes sense to see how it slips in, since it tends to be overused, creeping into the diet without being recognized as a contributor toward total fats.

Maybe you put:
1 teaspoon on hot oatmeal
1 teaspoon on a piece of toast
2 teaspoons on a sandwich at lunchtime
1 tablespoon on green beans at dinner
2 tablespoons in mashed potatoes, also at dinner

If you had spent the day measuring and counting, you'd see how much fat you had consumed in the form of margarine: 13 teaspoons, more than half a stick, in a single day. This does not account for additional fat you've ingested in salad dressing or mayonnaise, in cookies, crackers, or other snacks. It doesn't account for any fat you might have used in cooking a chicken breast, for example, let alone the fat found in the chicken breast itself. It doesn't leave room for any monounsaturated fats, such as olive or canola oil, which might actually have some health benefits. And yet those 13 teaspoons are the equivalent of 65 grams, something like a serving of that deadly red-eye gravy mentioned above. (If you are partial to math problems, check the Endnote[22] to see how this was worked out.) Fat adds up very, very quickly.

Using Fat in Recipes

Another example of the use of margarine can be found in baking. We've selected oatmeal cookies because they sound so wholesome. This genuine, bona fide recipe yields 48 cookies. It calls for:

2 1/2 cups oats
1 3/4 cups flour
2 eggs
1/2 cup granulated sugar
1 cup brown sugar
1 teaspoon baking soda
1 teaspoon vanilla
1/2 teaspoon salt
1 CUP MARGARINE

We'll spare you the blending and the beating and the adding and the mixing and the dropping-by-teaspoonful-on-greased-cookie-sheets. The bottom line is that our batch of cookies contains 1 cup (48 teaspoons) of margarine, or one teaspoon per cookie (5 grams). If they aren't burned, it wouldn't be hard to polish off 13 cookies, a baker's dozen, but look how much fat they contain: a grand total of 65 grams.

Sizing

Up

Fat

*Stick with
Jack Sprat,
not Jack
Sprat's wife,
in the
supermarket*

.

Putting It All Together

Remember Elvis's red-eye gravy? And the bits of margarine at meal times that added up to half a stick? And the 13 home-made oatmeal cookies? They have something in common, which is that they all contain about 65 grams of fat. You're not going to forget this number, because you'll see it on food labels everywhere. Here's why.

Believe it or not, there are researchers who have devoted their lives to figuring out The Big Picture, the limit to how much fat should be consumed each day, and 65 grams is the number they came up with, the number you'll see on those food labels. This may not exactly be your personal number, which depends on size and activity level, but it's in the ballpark. (If you want more information on determining your personal "fat limit," there are many, many texts available on the subject.[23])

Sixty-five grams, then, is a number that you need to be familiar with. It is MORE THAN ENOUGH FAT FOR AN ENTIRE DAY on a relatively low-fat diet, according to the food label. (In chapter eleven, "How To Use Food Labels To Select Low-fat Foods," you'll see that even 65 grams may be much too much for you, and why.) As it is, Americans have so much fat in their food that it's amazing they don't just slide out of bed in the morning. There are people who actually get close to half their day's calories from fat. The thinking is that if fat could be reduced to no more than 30 percent of a day's calories, people would also reduce the likelihood that they'd fall prey to the evils of heart disease. (The figure "30 percent" is getting a lot of press, and you may already have heard it tossed around.)

But there's no need to get all involved with numbers. Stick with Jack Sprat, not Jack Sprat's wife, in the supermarket.

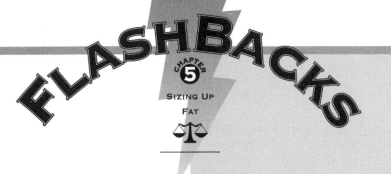

FLASHBACKS

CHAPTER
5

SIZING UP

FAT

☞ Remember that there are *5 grams of fat in 1 tea-spoon of oil.*

☞ **Sixty-five grams of fat is more than enough for an entire day.** Spread it throughout the day, rather than taking it all in at once (a serving of red-eye gravy, 13 cookies, whatever).

Chapter Six
Snacking

The Mindless Event

S NACKING is a common way for fat to creep into the diet, because fat is found in all sorts of packaged foods, from cookies and cakes to chips and crackers. It's too bad, but snack foods as we know and love them are associated with high fat and pleasure and chips and chocolate and cheese and dips and nachos. (Think of "junk food" as the contradiction in terms that it is.) You can probably conjure up one or two occasions when these things didn't appeal to you, but you'll probably also recall that you were in bed with a stomach virus at the time.

Snacking itself is not necessarily a bad thing (depending, of course, on what you snack on). That is, the body is designed for small, frequent meals. If you eat one or two large meals during the day, you are more likely to store fat; by distributing the calories throughout the day, you are less likely to gain weight. However, the body is not, repeat not, designed for small, frequent meals plus one or two big meals every day, which is what a lot of us have.

The trouble is, snacking becomes a kind of mindless event, a way to get through some of the shows that miraculously find their way onto the television screen. The mindlessness means that you won't be thinking about fat content and serving size, certainly not about your OPSS (Own Personal Serving Size), and it doesn't take much to go from OPSS to OOPS! Let's use Wheat Thins as an example of doing just that. (We've chosen Wheat Thins because one of us, the one with naturally curly hair, was more or less addicted to them in a former, higher fat, life.)

Say you sit down in front of the TV with a box of Wheat Thins and eat the whole box, and say you are compulsive enough that you counted them out as you were eating them. You'd know you just ate 160 crackers. Check that label and you'll see one serving is 16 crackers, but that your Own Personal Serving Size (OPSS) was, at least on this particular occasion, *ten times* that on the label.

How much fat are you getting? The label will tell you that there are

6 grams of fat per serving. Multiply that times your 10 servings, and you'll come to the unhappy realization that you've just consumed 60 grams of fat.

How could you have stopped yourself from eating the whole box of crackers? We've had a certain amount of success closing up the box and flinging it across the room. Being too lazy to get up and go after it, we don't eat any more crackers. We've also found it useful to throw the uneaten crackers into the garbage and cover them with coffee grounds. Even our beloved Wheat Thins are not all that appetizing in such a condition.

The Addiction

Snacking is complicated and food manufacturers know that. So maybe they use a little fun and a little humor to divert you from the issues. Take SMARTFOOD Popcorn, for example. It contains no artificial flavors or preservatives and comes "butter flavored" or "with WHITE cheddar cheese seasoning." Let's take a look at the cheddar cheese version.

Calling a food SMARTFOOD may be a clever marketing gimmick (since it is clearly not the food that is smart but the people who buy it), but we like to think that consumers aren't so naive as to judge a product by its name alone.

Or by its package. There is a pleasant irreverence on bags of SMART-FOOD Popcorn that can catch you off guard. Little testimonials, sent in by satisfied customers, are printed on the back of the bag. One such testimonial, in the form of a poem, begins, "I crave it every minute," and goes on to confess an inability to resist eating SMARTFOOD popcorn. Snacking, the addiction.

According to the label, the bag contains seven servings of about 1 3/4 cups each. We're here to tell you that there were 88 kernels in our one and three-quarters cups. How long does it take to eat those 88 kernels?

Snacking

Typical snack foods have little place in a low-fat diet.

Funny you should ask. It took one of us (the "perm person") four and a half minutes to consume them, working slowly and steadily, eating three to four kernels at a time. We all know that people often tend to eat popcorn quickly and steadily, and they may not stop eating after four and a half minutes. If you can't resist eating SMARTFOOD popcorn, if you just can't stay away from it, who knows? The whole bag may be your serving.

But there is the small matter of fat content. The label states that a 1 3/4-cup serving contains 10 grams of fat (and we can see from the label that more than half the calories in each serving come from fat). So if you are addicted enough to eat the whole bag, all seven servings just for you, that's 70 grams of fat. You might just as well sit down and eat half a stick of margarine. Yummy-yum? We don't think so.

Where does this leave us? The truth is that typical snack foods have limited usefulness, very limited usefulness, on a low-fat diet.

Snacking for the Chocoholic And the Chipsoholic

We've been suggesting healthy snacks. But what if you want chocolate, crave chocolate, ABSOLUTELY HAVE TO HAVE CHOCOLATE? Make a cup of Alba hot cocoa, or add Hershey's syrup to skim milk and have a glass of fat-free chocolate milk. If this sounds too healthy, have a fat-free Fudgsicle, which will give you the flavor (but not the fat) of chocolate. Or make a sundae with nonfat frozen yogurt and that same Hershey's syrup.

If these fat-free versions of chocolate don't satisfy your cravings, stick to dark rather than milk chocolate. Cocoa butter (found in dark chocolate) appears to be less harmful than butterfat (found in milk chocolate). But you'll have to read labels to make sure the chocolate you are buying does not contain butterfat. Remember, too, that where fat is concerned, serving size becomes important, so share some of that chocolate with your very best friends.

And what if you crave potato chips, cannot imagine life without that fatty snack? First of all, you might come across one of the new, fat-free versions. But there's no getting around it, these don't taste like high-fat chips. If that's what you are craving, then take an occasional fat holiday. Factor the chips into your diet, using your fat for the day in snack form. This will mean eating no additional fat that day and making sure to eat plenty of starches, plenty of fresh fruits and vegetables, and putting a fat-free dressing on your salad in order to allow for fatty snacks.

You have to plan for this. If you are going out to eat, or if food will otherwise be out of your control one day, don't pick that day to consume your day's fat in potato chips. And, needless to say, you won't eat unlimited quantities of chips. You'll read the label, be shocked to see how much fat is in them, and then figure out what serving size will fit into The Big Picture of total daily fat. A 6-ounce bag of chips contains *60 grams of fat*, otherwise known as "enough fat for the entire day."

Plan, plan, plan.

The Fat-Free Chocolate-Covered Creme-Filled Mini-Cakes Diet

T he latest trend in snacking is getting the fat out, and we most certainly have the technology to do it. Liposuction, the popular surgical technique that sucks the fat out of thighs and other parts of the body where it is deemed undesirable, is now being used on food. Or something like liposuction, anyway. Food manufacturers, ever anxious to jump on a lucrative bandwagon, even if it's a health-

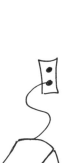

Snacking

"Fat free" doesn't equal "calorie free."

oriented one, are flooding the market with fat-free versions of everything they can get their hands on.

What this means is that, if your sole focus is on lowering fat, watch out. You might very well find yourself on the *Fat-Free Chocolate-Covered Creme-Filled Mini-Cakes Diet.* If, as they say, "you are what you eat," you could be in trouble.

It's a fat-free diet all right. Fat free and sweet. Very seductive. If your aim is to lower fat, you might think that Fat-Free Chocolate-Covered Creme-Filled Mini-Cakes would be just the thing to have at breakfast. And again at lunch. And at snack time, too.

Oh, by the way, did we mention that the Fat-Free Chocolate-Covered Creme-Filled Mini-Cakes Diet is a weight-*gain* diet? That "fat free" doesn't equal "calorie free"? And that great minds are asking: No fiber, no fat, no vitamins, no minerals – what in the world is this?

If you have never eaten Fat-Free Chocolate-Covered Creme-Filled Mini-Cakes, you might want to know that not everyone falls in love with them. Plenty of people find that taking out the fat has made them chewy and hyper-sweet, with a lingering taste that even strong, black coffee doesn't wash away. Then again, if you want to have one piece of cake and taste it for the rest of the day, this could be for you.

One man, whose birthday cake was made from the stuff, blew out the candles, ate the first piece, and said, barely containing his disappointment, "Why didn't you just sing 'Birthday to You'?" Then the ice cream was served. Well, it wasn't exactly ice cream. It wasn't ice milk, either. It was . . . it was . . . "frozen dessert."

Fat-Free Chocolate-Covered Creme-Filled Mini-Cakes are not the answer to getting the fat out. Real food is vastly preferable, so look first for starches with no added fat, look carefully at starches with added fat, and look with suspicion at starches from which the fat has been liposuctioned.

Smart Snacking

someone could make a lot of money with a line of healthy snack foods. They could be called "Sound Bites," a take-off on the media term you hear all the time. Or maybe Good-4-U-Snax –"Snack your way to a healthier you!" There they'd be, an array of packages you could put on your shelf, open whenever you felt like a snack, and know that you were getting a nutritious, low-fat or nonfat snack that, not incidentally, tasted absolutely wonderful. Trouble is, what you'd find when you opened up those Good-4-U-Snax would be six fat-free saltines, an apple, and a glass of skim milk staring up at you. Not exactly what you had in mind, is it?

Luckily, Chocolate-Covered Creme-Filled Mini-Cakes are not the only snacks that have come on the market with "FAT FREE" in banner letters across the package. There are others that, while not exactly "Good-4-U," come a lot closer than those Fat-Free Chocolate-Covered Creme-Filled Mini-Cakes do. They are made from starches such as corn or rice or potatoes (like the fat-free potato chips mentioned a minute ago), and become crispy snacks without the addition of fat.

Sometimes, though, the words "FAT FREE" appear big and bold on the package, but there is fat on the Ingredient List. How can this be? The answer is simply that so little fat was used in processing that the product is considered fat free. ("Fat free," according to the label law, means there is less than half a gram of fat in one serving.) However, if the fat listed is hydrogenated or partially hydrogenated, find another snack. Even in small quantities, hydrogenated fat is to be avoided.

Still, if you want less fat in your diet and at the same time you want to eat real food, you'll have to think about snacking the way you think about eating in general. Try filling up with something starchy (go back and check out the Pyramid of Starches) like bread or sourdough pretzels (salted or unsalted depending on sodium restrictions, and check the label to be sure they are fat free), even a bowl of cereal with skim milk. Popcorn is a good choice, but make sure you air-pop it. Even microwave

Avoid snacks containing hydrogenated fat.

Snacking

popcorn is – surprise, surprise! – high in fat, especially when you take your OPSS (Own Personal Serving Size) into account.

IF YOU WANT TO BE A LITTLE INVENTIVE

Try leftover new potatoes or corn on the cob. Nabisco makes fat-free saltines; Health Valley makes fat-free crackers; Guiltless Gourmet makes No Oil Tortilla chips, all of which go nicely with salsa or with Guiltless Gourmet's fat-free bean dips. New products are coming on the market constantly, so keep your eyes open and see what's around. Starches have the enormous advantage of making you feel satisfied.

Smart Snacking: The Plan of Attack

In case you haven't noticed, snacking and socializing go hand in hand. You go to the movies, you snack. (Buttered popcorn? Shoebox-size box of Milk Duds?) You take a break at work, you snack, maybe hit the vending machines. (Peanut butter crackers? Potato chips?)

You can still snack and socialize; it's just that your snacks will be different. If you know where you spend your time, you can find out in advance where you can get low-fat snacks. In other words, know your territory. This thinking applies whether you are socializing or not. If you spend time in the mall, say, know where you can buy nonfat frozen yogurt, or a fancy coffee or tea. If you pass convenience stores each day, know which ones sell bagels and fresh fruit and fruit-flavored seltzer. (Seltzer? Yes, because if you feel hungry, you might really be thirsty! Strange but true, maybe, but a glass of water often takes care of "hunger.") If you're working in an office building, know what time the cafeteria opens so you don't have to rely on those vending machines.

We've said it before, we'll say it again: Real food is vastly preferable, so that's what to look for when you feel like snacking.

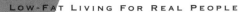

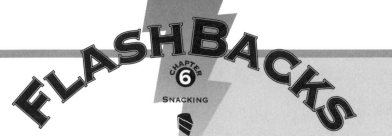

CHAPTER
6
SNACKING

☞ **Plan snacks carefully and SNACK SMART!**
Because snacking is a mindless event, you can take in a lot of fat very quickly. It doesn't take much to go from OPSS to OOPS!

☞ **Check out the Pyramid of Starches.**
Eat real food–starches–for snacks.

☞ **Good snack choices:**
Fat-free bagel, apple, banana, raw carrot
Guiltless Gourmet No Oil Tortilla Chips (with fat-free bean dip or salsa)
Snyder's of Hanover Sourdough Pretzels (unsalted, if you are trying to eat less salt)

☞ **If you crave chocolate:**
Try a fat-free Fudgsicle.
Try nonfat frozen yogurt with Hershey's syrup.
Try Alba hot cocoa.

☞ The Fat-Free Chocolate-Covered-Creme-Filled-Mini-Cakes Diet sounds good but isn't, so –
Look first for starches with no added fat.
Look carefully at starches with added fat.
Look with suspicion at starches from which the fat has been "liposuctioned."

☞ **"Fat free" isn't "calorie free."**

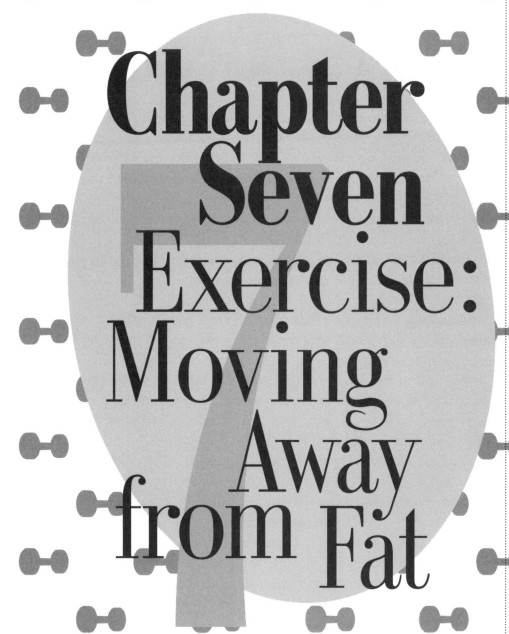

Chapter Seven
Exercise: Moving Away from Fat

Exercise:

Moving Away

from Fat

Making A Case For Exercise

I f you eat too much food, even fat-free food, you'll find yourself putting on weight, the traditional reason for exercising. Traditional, but not only. Muscles work better when they are used, and the heart is a muscle, the "muscle of choice" in this case. When you get your blood flowing, you exercise your heart. (Before making changes in your activity level, you should, of course, check with your doctor.)

Like a lot of people, you may feel that "exercise" amounts to putting forth a major effort just in order to sweat, shower, and change your clothes in the middle of the day. It means stopping whatever you are doing, going to the gym (alias "health club") and "working out" surrounded by other people who are working out and apparently having a wonderful time (are they hired for this, or what?), their already-perfect bodies clad in merciless exercise outfits that offer no hiding places for unsightly bulges. Going to the gym means riding a bike that doesn't go anywhere, taking a long walk on a short treadmill, and climbing stairs that stay put.

Did Cave Man go out to exercise? Or, for that matter, Cave Woman? Well, yes, as a matter of fact, but they didn't call it that, and they certainly didn't go to a gym to do it. Exercise was built into their lives, since common, everyday activities, like grocery shopping, were pretty arduous back then. By contrast, our lives are often physically undemanding, and so we compartmentalize exercise, give it a special time of day, a special name, and buy special clothes to wear when we are doing it. But there is another way to stay (or become) physically fit, without resorting to exercise videos and health clubs and spandex.

Exercise: The "Fun" Part

In your search for The Ideal Exercise, keep in mind that you don't have to call it "exercise." In some circles, the term "physical activity" has come into vogue. Keep in mind as well: ❶ nontraditional forms of aerobic activity are fine; ❷ you have to do whatever it is regularly – three to four times a week should be about right; ❸ it's okay to enjoy yourself. Anything goes, as long as it keeps you moving vigorously for twenty to thirty minutes. You'll know you have selected the perfect activity for yourself when you don't realize that the allotted time has passed.

Why nontraditional aerobic activity? Because the workout aspect is incidental to the pleasure of performing the activity. If you like doing something, you'll do it, and that's the key, not just talk about it, but do it, and do it regularly. (A friend of ours tells us that he runs "three miles *a time*." He may run regularly, but apparently he doesn't run often. Still, he's clever. We'll give him that.)

Say you love rowing a boat. Great! But how often can you do it? If you have ready access to a rowboat (not to mention water), you're all set. Or say you love conducting an orchestra. Also great! But if you can only occasionally get to a boat – or an orchestra – well, that brings up something we should discuss.

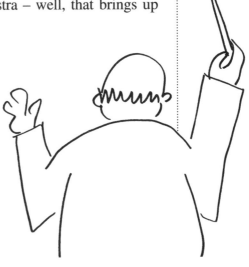

Variety:
Also the Spice of Exercise

You can vary your activities. The easiest in terms of convenience, accessibility, and necessary equipment, is walking. So maybe you take a good, brisk walk in the early morning several times a week. But if you're bored, try other aerobic activities from time to time, like dancing. (Aerobic activity makes your heart beat faster, makes you breathe harder, makes you take in more oxygen.)

Dancing? Yes, dancing. It can be one of the great nontraditional aerobic workouts going. Dancing can be enjoyed alone or with a partner, and there are dances to suit almost everyone, whether young and tired or old and vigorous. Pick your style.

Unlike aerobics classes, the object of which is to finish (". . . five and four and three and two and one!"), the object of dance is to continue. There is whirling, gyrating, turning, bending, reaching, twisting, arms and legs moving continuously to music, and the music keeps you going, catches you up so that you don't think about time, don't think about anything at all, hypnotized as you are by repetitive movements, you just keep going, you don't stop, no one stops, as long as the music is playing.

Now it just may be that you like going to a gym, that your personal "Stairway to Heaven" is a stair-climbing machine, and you don't think of it as a set of stairs that stays put. Maybe you like rowing, but you prefer a rowing machine to a boat on a lake. Maybe you'd rather do your cross-country skiing indoors, where it's warm, using a device built for exactly that. Of course that's fine, and you'll have plenty of company.

But if you hate the idea of working out, let alone changing your clothes to do so, then try something – anything! – else. Your body will love you for it.

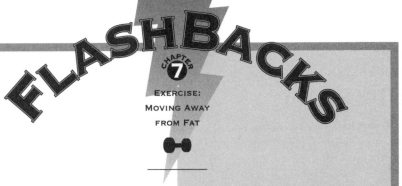

FLASHBACKS

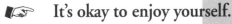

👉 **It's okay to enjoy yourself.**

👉 **Exercise regularly,** about three to four times a week.

👉 **Sustain activity for about twenty to thirty minutes.**

👉 **Choose the perfect activity for yourself.** You'll know it is because you won't realize that the allotted time has passed.

Chapter Eight
Strategies for Eating Out

Strategies

for

Eating Out

Eating in Restaurants: Replacing Fat Gram Counters with Common Sense

Actually there are two ways to eat out: in a restaurant and at someone's house. While the restaurant is more expensive, it's a lot easier to deal with, assuming that it's one where the food is carefully cooked to order. Unfortunately this is not true of "all you can eat" places, where everything is already prepared when you arrive, and they are just waiting to see how much you really can put away. Portions tend to be enormous, which translates into an unacceptable amount of fat.

When you eat out, it's hard to know just how much fat you're getting in your food. However, if you keep your fat intake under control the rest of the day, then, when you go to a restaurant, all you'll have to do is order sensibly, and you're about to see how to do that. You won't have to burden yourself with one of those fat gram counters you see everywhere, either. Instead of sitting there thumbing through a book, the way you do when you're visiting a foreign country where you don't speak the language, you'll be free to enjoy your meal – which is, after all, the whole point.

Restaurants: Out with Friends

Sometimes life has a way of working out. By the time you have concluded that Twinkies are not one of the basic food groups (well, not part of the Pyramid), you've reached the point where you no longer have to be one of the crowd, ordering what everyone else orders, never mind if their taste runs to foods so rich and heavy that you have to sign a medical release before you consume them. On the other hand, if you still want to have friends, it might be better not to point out their poor food choices just now. Soon enough your habits will begin to show, and you'll find that as they start in on an enormous slab of fatty roast beef, they'll say something like, "Boy, I haven't eaten meat in six months!" Better not mention that they said that last week, and the week before, too, come to think of it. Watching you eat may be making them feel guilty.

And they may become "friendly enemies," people who mean well when they urge you to eat something that won't hurt "just this once."

Just this once. Think about that for a minute. In theory, just this once wouldn't matter, of course. But in practice, it would be possible to have 365 unacceptable dishes per year (366 on leap year) and that could spell trouble. Note that these foods may still crop up on special occasions, but that a "special occasion" involves more than merely going out for dinner. Think "Birthday with a Zero in It"; think "Major Anniversary"; think "Unbelievable Job Promotion."

IF YOU EAT AT RESTAURANTS FREQUENTLY, YOU CANNOT CONSIDER EVERY RESTAURANT MEAL A SPECIAL EVENT. It is merely a convenience, a chance to have a meal without the nuisance of preparing it. When delicious but fatty foods come your way, which they will routinely if you're eating in restaurants, you'll have to be strong about this: Stand pat, stand firm, stand up for your rights. This may come in the form of a gentle shake of the head (as in "No, thank you"), or a firm "No, thank you."

Tips on How to Order

Study the menu. Think "no cream, no cheese, no butter." Order foods that are broiled or grilled rather than fried, passing up things like deep fried fat, tempting though they may be, and popular, too, heaven knows. Avoid dishes that are described as "pan-fried," "crispy," "au gratin" (with cheese), "Parmesan" (with Parmesan cheese), and "scalloped" or "escalloped" (sounds like scallops are involved, but most often it is something that finds itself awash in a rich sauce).

When the server comes to take your order, you might consider saying that you are on a "medical diet." Since restaurants customarily consider it bad for business when a patron keels over during the main course, they

Think:
no cream
no cheese
no butter

Strategies

for

Eating Out

*Ask to have
vegetables
rinsed with
boiling
water.*

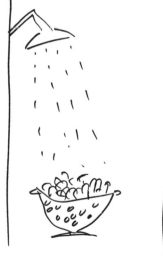

will be much more likely to comply with your wishes.

You are about to make a number of demands, but at the same time, you don't want to appear to be demanding. One woman we know has gone to the extreme, and asks so gently and so quietly that hers is often the order that never finds its way to the kitchen. You can be more demanding than that. You have a right to be. It's your own health and well-being, and you can be cheerful but firm in requesting certain things.

Ask how various dishes are prepared. Well-educated restaurants provide their servers with specific information, and they will, if necessary, ask the chef for more details. The server is, in other words, your link to the kitchen.

Ask for your salad with the dressing on the side, too. Many a server will nod vigorously when you do because it's such a common request. And while you're at it, select a dressing that is not one of those thick, creamy ones. An oil and vinegar dressing is better, and best of all is simply to ask for the oil and vinegar so that you can make your own dressing and use less oil.

Ask that butter be left off (even a grilled entrée may arrive swimming in butter that has been put on top after it's cooked) and that sauces be served on the side. Rather than immediately dumping the sauce onto your food, try using just a little bit for flavor, maybe dipping the fork in it so that you get a taste with the food. This is called taking charge of your life.

Ask, too, how the vegetables are prepared. If preparation involves the use of olive oil, you can ask them to go easy. If preparation involves butter or rich sauces, you can ask to have the vegetables steamed. Maybe the server will tell you sorry, it's too late, they're made in advance, in which case simply ask if they could be put into a colander and rinsed with boiling water.

Once your order has been placed, your conversation with the server may not be over. In spite of your best efforts, when your food arrives, it might not be exactly what you asked for.

◆　　◆　　◆　　◆

In the old days, when you went to a restaurant with a group of people and your order came out well done when you'd asked for it rare, well, maybe you said something and maybe you didn't. It might have been the case that only the members of your party who had the word "obnoxious" tattooed on their foreheads would think of sending back their food, a gesture that was perceived as unpleasant, disruptive, and, in general, antisocial.

Now you have more at stake. If there is something the matter with your order, you'll want to say so. There are, of course, ways to do this. A not so fine line exists between "assertive" and "aggressive"; assertive is the way to go. Think of this as taking care of yourself, rather than an attempt to win the Most Offensive award.

You don't have to make a big deal of the fact that even though you asked for no butter, you could spot your order shimmering at twenty paces. You simply say quietly to the server, "I'm sorry to have to ask you to take this back, but I did order it without butter." There's no need to be embarrassed. If those in your group elect to make a major production out of this, then they, not you, deserve to be embarrassed.

Salad Bars

A few words about salad bars. They get a lot of mileage out of their name. If they were called, say, "glop stops," they wouldn't attract much business. But, in fact, glop stops is a great deal more descriptive of what they really are.

The average salad bar has a large bowl of lettuce, lying on top of which is a pair of tongs, cleverly designed so that when you pick up a generous portion of lettuce leaves, most of them fall back into the bowl before you can get them on your plate. And then there are all those people behind you in line, and, well, you just have to keep moving.

What you move on to are a series of cold concoctions that are, more often than not, loaded with fat and calories. You'll find potato salad, cole slaw, macaroni salad in a thick oil dressing. You'll find chopped egg (it's the yolks that contain fat, but if you try to pick out the whites here, you'll cause a riot), grated cheese (contains fat), mushrooms soaking in oil, and more. You'll also find tomatoes, fresh mushrooms, cucumbers, onions, peppers, pickled beets, and other typical salad ingredients. Here you are,

"I'm sorry to have to ask you to take this back, but I did order it without butter."

Strategies

for

Eating Out

As a rule, the heavier the salad bar item, the higher the fat content.

holding up the line, and you have to think fast. In fact, it's quite simple. As a rule, the heavier the salad bar item, the higher the fat content (with the exception of carrots and beets). Think what you'd put in ye olde salade bowle if you were fixing an ordinary salad at home, go forth, and do likewise.

At the end of the bar you'll see vats of various salad dressings, sometimes identified, sometimes not, and even when they are identified you might not realize it because the signs are sitting on top of the plastic cover of the salad bar, not exactly in your line of sight. The thicker dressings come in creamy white, tan, even pink. There is probably a brown, oil-based dressing there, too. Whatever their color, THESE DRESSINGS ARE FULL OF FAT, unless they are labeled "fat free." Incidentally, those long-handled ladles that hang over the edge of the dressing containers hold two tablespoons of dressing, which, if labeled, would announce the sad fact that *they contain close to 20 grams of fat.*

The dressings can be a fine addition to a salad, greatly improving the chances that you'll eat and enjoy it. So use some, not a lot, maybe about one fourth of a ladleful.

Better to use the oil and vinegar that you'll find in the two little bottles sure to be around there someplace. Then (okay, this is asking a lot) just splash some vinegar on top and feel incredibly virtuous.

Bread and Butter

While you're waiting for your food to come, you'll notice that bread (or rolls) and butter have been brought to the table. Many times they take the form of buttery rolls and garlic bread. It is sort of a knee-jerk reaction to consume large portions while you have a nice conversation and perhaps a glass of wine.

Ask the server for plain bread, and eat it without the butter that will be served attractively in little pots, or in little candy shapes, or in a ball that looks like a scoop of ice cream. If you are in the habit of using butter, you'll probably want to put it out of arm's reach, admittedly not easy when you consider the size of some of the tables in restaurants these days. The idea is to be fully aware of what you're eating, rather than awaken from a trance to find that you aren't very hungry, what with that entire loaf of garlic bread in your stomach.

Serving Size

You really have no control over restaurant serving sizes. You take what you get, and it's usually more than you need in the way of meat/poultry/fish. If it tastes good, you eat all of it. Even if it doesn't taste wonderful, the old tapes play in your head – "Clean your plate! People are starving all over the world!" – and you finish anyway.

There are options. You can divide the portion and ask to have part of it wrapped to take home. You can offer some to others in your group. If neither of these works (maybe you're on your way to a party and don't want to leave food sitting in the car half the night; maybe there are no takers for your leftovers), you have a last resort. We've tried it and guarantee that it works. (See box.)

> **THE LAST RESORT:**
>
> Pick up the salt shaker and, with a last look around, put so much salt on the meat/poultry/fish that it becomes inedible. That way, you won't sit there and pick, pick, pick until you suddenly notice that you've eaten the whole thing, even though you had no intention of doing so. A no-fail way to limit serving size.

Dessert

You don't need to read here that fresh fruit is the best possible dessert pick because you already know that. If you absolutely must have a sweet dessert, make it something like fruit pie, but not à la mode. Remember that "la mode" – the fashion – these days is to cut down on things like ice cream. See if you can get someone to split a piece of pie with you. That way, unless you are on the attack, you will eat only half. You'll eat even less if your companion is on the attack. If you can manage to avoid eating the crust, the fattiest part of the pie, so much the better. Otherwise, try eating just half of it.

The ever-popular dessert tray makes life all the more difficult because you can see what you're missing, and that's no accident. Apparently the word is out that restaurant patrons who see "mocha whipped cream torte" printed on a menu may pass it up, but they may not be able to resist upon seeing the dessert itself. The server arrives with the dessert tray and describes, in such detail that you can feel yourself gaining weight just by listening to each delectable offering. But do your best to stay away from rich pastries and other creamy things, which are nothing more than morsels (granted, tasty morsels) of fat and calories – and what most people imagine when the word "dessert" comes into the conversation. Instead, try one of the fruit ices that are popular, so popular, in fact, that they are being called "sorbets," which just goes to show how classy things sound in French. Frequently they are homemade and are a refreshing end to the meal.

> ### BE CREATIVE
>
> If there is a raspberry purée over the chocolate cheesecake, and they also offer fresh straw-berries, ask if you might have strawberries with the raspberry purée. Or, if they have no fruit listed, ask. It may be available as an appetizer and they will serve it to you for dessert.

An old diet expression says, "A minute on the lips, a lifetime on the hips." That thinking works here, too. If you give in and eat that rich, creamy, chocolate dessert, it's gone in a minute, but the effects linger in your body. The rhyme may be lost, but the idea isn't. And it's not just your hips, it's your heart.

Coffee and Tea

If you like a good cup of coffee or fragrant tea and must lighten it, ask for milk instead of cream. Make it low-fat milk if they have it, which they probably won't, but if enough people ask for it, you can be sure they'll get it eventually. Don't be fooled into thinking that nondairy creamers are better; their big advantage is to shopkeepers since they don't spoil, but they may contain a lot of fat.

A glass of sparkling water with a lemon or lime wedge also makes a nice ending for the meal. If it is served in one of those great-looking glasses that restaurants are investing in, it will seem to taste all the better.

Lunch

When you are really and truly watching your food intake, one of the day-to-day problems you will face is lunch. Of course you've always thought of lunch as a meal, not a problem, but it can be both a meal and a problem.

The difficulty comes when you work in an office and lunch consists of a fast bite somewhere. Since fast bites are generally high in fat, the solution is to carry your lunch with you.

Now it may well be that the last time you carried your lunch it was in a lunch box with your favorite cartoon character painted all over it, and a small thermos bottle tucked inside it whose glass liner broke and had to be replaced every week. (Could it have been because you played catch with it on the school bus?)

If you're feeling a little crazy, you might buy yourself a new lunch box. Lunch boxes are still around, but the thermos bottles have an unbreakable plastic lining. Your old favorite cartoon friends may be gone, but you'll find an enormous selection of possible replacements.

Undoubtedly it has already occurred to you that you do not need a lunch box in order to carry your lunch. You can use anything from a brown bag (simple but nice) to an attaché case (upscale and trendy). The issue is what to take in it.

To a great extent, this will depend on where you are going to be doing your eating. If you'll be staying at your desk, is there a microwave oven nearby? This would allow you to pack leftovers from last night's dinner; they could be reheated quickly and easily. If you have no access to a microwave, or if you are of the persuasion that you'll glow in the dark if you get too close to one, think "cold food." Maybe those same leftovers.

Lunch: Sandwiches

The most obvious cold lunch is a sandwich and the flat, round pocket bread known as pita is one possible bread choice. Widely available in supermarkets, this no-fat-added bread comes in white and whole wheat, and in two sizes, the larger of which is easier to use for sand-

Strategies

for

Eating Out

wiches. If you cut the bread in half, you have two half-circles with an opening, a pocket, exposed. Now you have only to decide how to fill it.

You might make a tuna salad using one of those little cans of water-packed, rather than oil-packed, tuna. The two varieties sit side by side on your grocer's shelf, and you just have to make sure you pick up the right one. If you've still got some oil-packed tuna in your cupboard, or if you find that you grabbed the wrong one after all, dump it into a strainer and run cold water over it. You'll get rid of most of the oil.

Drain the tuna as you would do normally, and mix it with chopped onion or peppers, maybe some shredded carrot and a bit of horseradish for spice, whatever you like. (Better skip the onions if you've got a big post-lunch meeting scheduled.) Instead of using mayonnaise, or even so-called "lite" mayonnaise, try a bit of mustard (one that contains no oil) mixed with nonfat yogurt (see recipe for Yogurt-Mustard Sauce, page 177. Or see recipe for Crunchy Tuna Salad, page 149).

Now stuff some romaine lettuce into the pita – it fits more easily if you first cut it up or pull it apart – add the tuna, and you're all set.

> ### FOR A REAL TREAT
> Instead of tuna, try a bit of cold salmon from last night's Salmon Cooked in Foil (see recipe, page 146) or maybe some leftover Grilled Turkey (see recipe, page 142).

You can make a salad sandwich by cutting up any vegetables you like – carrots, celery, radishes, cucumbers, peppers, onions, tomatoes, and so on. (Is it true that tomatoes are really fruits? Inquiring minds want to know.) You could put in marinated beans and vegetables (see recipe for Marinated Beans and Vegetables, page 167). Sprouts are delicious with this. Should you be under the impression that sprouts are for antiestablishment-vegetarian-hippie types, guess again. They are very tasty and add a nice texture to the contents of the sandwich. (You can grow sprouts or buy them at the supermarket. Once upon a time, we did the former. Now we do the latter.) Stuff the mixture into the pita, and drizzle over it that Yogurt-Mustard Sauce mentioned a minute ago.

You can always use fat-free bagels. "A sandwich from a bagel?" you are thinking. If that sounds just a little too Whopper-sized for you, consider eating a salad with a bagel on the side. You can keep bagels on hand in the freezer. (Hint: Slice them before freezing. Slicing a frozen bagel is so difficult and dangerous that it could be an Olympic event.)

Eating Out for Breakfast

You may have noticed that eating out for breakfast hasn't been discussed. The brutal fact is that breakfast foods tend to be high, often very high, in fat: eggs, bacon, sausage, et cetera, et cetera, et cetera. If you find yourself eating breakfast in a restaurant, you can always order oatmeal, but not everyone considers it a big treat. If you want More Traditional Breakfast Fare, you can cut your losses by ordering pancakes or waffles without that dollop of butter on top, and then use syrup. In fact, pancakes or waffles are a better choice than muffins, croissants, and doughnuts, which are generally loaded with fat.

Another possibility is to order an egg substitute or an egg white omelet. This can then be filled with peppers, mushrooms, tomatoes, onions, whatever, but not cheese. It's worth keeping in mind that restaurants offering egg white omelets have to do something with the yolks, and chances are extremely good that what they do with them is to add them to the regular omelet mixture, thereby increasing the fat content of those omelets.

Restaurants frequently use plastic squeeze bottles of margarine and squirt it in pans and on the grill when they prepare food. Obviously this adds a lot of fat to whatever food is cooked there. So you'll want to ask that your omelet be prepared without fat on the grill. This won't affect preparation, because the grill is already seasoned and the omelet won't stick.

Order a bagel, an English muffin, or toast, dry (no butter or margarine), and spread it with jam or honey.

Pancakes or waffles (without butter) are a better choice than muffins, croissants, and doughnuts.

Strategies

for

Eating Out

Eating at Someone's House

At a restaurant you can order whatever you want, which wouldn't go over very well at a dinner party, where the custom is to eat the food you're served, fat and all.

However, friends will take notice if you have developed a distinctive eating style. The fact that it is your chief subject of conversation may have something to do with it. If you were a vegetarian, a friend inviting you to a small dinner party would probably have you in mind when the menu was planned, and the same holds true here.

Yes, if this is just a few good friends getting together, you'll do fine. For one thing, your host may run the menu by you when the invitation is extended. For another, you can make simple requests at that time: Might some dressing be kept aside for your salad, so that you can add it yourself? And might some bread be left unbuttered for you? Then, too, you can offer to bring dessert, and bring a low-fat one.

Big Parties

The problem is with big parties, huge parties, weddings, and the key is to eat first. That's right, you're on your way out to dinner but you eat before you go. There's no need to sit down to a full-course meal, or to use a cloth napkin, but the idea is that you shouldn't be hungry when you get to this food fest. It's much easier to turn down the fried cheese balls being passed when you aren't in the first stages of starvation.

Life is a little easier if this is a buffet. You can take what you want and be spared that "pushing around" thing we all learned to do when we were kids and our plates were contaminated by peas.

Anyway, if the fare is spread out before you at a buffet table, count yourself lucky. And if someone is serving, so much the better, because you can ask casually what in the world this stuff is.

But there are those elegant dinner parties where the food is passed to you at the table, and you help yourself, putting it on a dinner plate the size of a

Have something to eat before going to big parties.

sombrero. Here comes the crab in cream sauce, the beef already coated with bearnaise sauce, the broccoli lost in hollandaise sauce. Here are the potatoes with butter and cheese, the already buttered rolls. It's lonely at the top.

But forge ahead as best you can, keeping in mind that you have to live in this world. You can take small portions, claiming that you spoiled your appetite by eating too many of those delicious – what were they? Oh, yes, of course! – fried cheese balls. Help yourself to a little bit of a couple of things, and surreptitiously scrape off as much of the sauce as you can manage without appearing to be playing with your food. Forget the rolls.

Dessert will undoubtedly be some rich something, and if you can bear to turn it down, do. If not, try to eat just a bit of it, and focus on what is sure to be the best cup of coffee since the Folger's people first pawned off instant coffee on unsuspecting restaurant patrons.

Develop a secret smile that you can use when other guests marvel at how little you eat. You, of course, are stuffed to the gills, having eaten at home, and you've had some extra goodies at this party.

Business Lunches and Dinners

There are times when your work involves a meal with a lot of other people, and the food has been ordered ahead of time. Maybe you had a little input ("Please check one: Chicken with Cream Sauce, Fried Fish Fillet"), but you understandably feel as though the food is pretty much out of your control at this point.

Not true! When you find that you'll be going to a restaurant or hotel for a meeting, don't be afraid to call ahead, speak to the catering department, and simply explain the situation. Most likely you'll be pleasantly surprised to find that the kitchen will be very accommodating, and will modify the menu to suit your needs.

Fast Food

A fast word on fast food restaurants. They boast an enormous wall menu that offers very little in the way of low-fat foods. Fish, normally considered low in fat, is not among them, being almost imvariably breaded and fried. Here are your choices:

Don't be afraid to call ahead and speak to the catering department.

Strategies

for

Eating Out

- Grilled, not breaded, chicken sandwich (plain, not deluxe)
- Junior hamburger (3 ounces, and hold the creamy sauces, cheese, et cetera)
- Grilled chicken/salad

Speaking of salad, the dressing comes in a little packet made of a material that is almost impossible to tear open. Which turns out to be just as well, because, unless the dressing is low fat or fat free, you're better off using none at all. One tiny packet contains up to 40 grams of fat, the equivalent of one third of a stick of margarine.

What else can you find to eat? Potatoes, but not fries. A baked potato is fine (if they have it), but order it plain; the fat hangs out in the toppings. Probably the closest thing you'll find to a vegetable is a side salad, not an interesting one at that, and you've just read the bad news about the dressing.

Pizza is another type of fast food that is high in fat, thanks to the meat, the cheese, and the oil. However, many places will make you a meatless, no-cheese pizza, easy on the oil.

It's worth taking the time to find fast food places that offer low-fat choices. Once you've found them, they'll be yours forever.

For the Healthy Traveler

I n today's busy world, it is essential that you not get so hungry that you grab anything handy, loaded with fat though it may be. When you are hungry, your goal is simply to fill your stomach, and only later do you reconsider, and rue, what you had to eat. It's a shame to fill yourself with fat-laden food that, most likely, doesn't taste very good anyway.

When you are traveling, you need something to tide you over until you can get some real food. If, say, you are traveling by airplane, take a couple of fat-free bagels, as well as apples or bananas, along for the ride. Chances are that it will be a long time until food service, and you'll have a good, filling, not particularly messy snack to munch on. Then, when the airline "food" (the term is used loosely) finally arrives, you won't be forced to eat it just because you are so hungry you're ready to eat the seat in front of you. Instead you can pick and choose from your food tray.

If, say, you are traveling by airplane, take a couple of fat-free bagels, as well as apples or bananas, along for the ride.

There will probably be a salad (try to go easy on the dressing), and a roll, which you can eat without butter (or whatever "spread" they offer, congratulating themselves for avoiding butter).

If the airline food falls into the "inedible" category, you can whip out a package of fat-free dehydrated soup (tasty soups are made by Nile Spice, Fantastic Foods, and Knorr, for example). It comes packaged in such a way that you add hot water (ask for some when the beverage service comes around) and eat it directly from the container the soup comes in. Handy. Disposable. Give it a try.

If you give them at least twenty-four hours' notice, airlines will provide a "special meal" for you. Your best bet is to request a diabetic meal (yes! really!) or a fresh fruit plate, tastier than the "low-fat" meals offered. We should mention that we have had a fair amount of experience with special meals that somehow never materialized, so don't assume you'll get one even if you requested it. ("When exactly did you order the meal?" we've been asked by the flight attendant. Were we paranoid in thinking she imagined herself in the company of a pathological liar?)

Maybe you are traveling to another country, where you'll be eating in restaurants. You might not be able to read the menu, and if you can't read it, you probably can't talk to the server, either. Here are some tips so you can at least steer clear of saturated fat:

HOW TO SAY, "PLEASE – NO CREAM, NO CHEESE, NO BUTTER," IN FOUR LANGUAGES.

FRENCH: S'il vous plaît ["seel voo play"]–sans ["sahn"] crème ["crem"], sans ["sahn"] fromage ["fro-mahj"], sans ["sahn"] beurre ["burr"].

SPANISH: Por favor ["poor fa-vour"]–sin ["sing"] crema ["crema"], sin ["sing"] queso ["kay-so"], sin ["sing"] mantequilla ["man-te-key-a"].

GERMAN: Bitte ["bit-uh"]–keine ["kine-uh"] Sahne ["sa-nuh"], kein ["kine"] Käse ["kayz-uh"], keine ["kine-uh"] Butter ["boot-er"].

ITALIAN: Per ["pair"] favore ["fa-vor-ay"]–niente ["nee-en-tay"] crema ["cray-ma"], niente ["nee-en-tay"] formaggio ["for-mah-jo"], niente ["nee-en-tay"] burro ["boor-o"].

Strategies

for

Eating Out

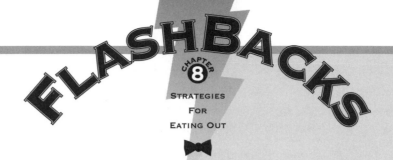

FLASHBACKS

CHAPTER 8

STRATEGIES
FOR
EATING OUT

☞ Take lunch to work.

☞ **If you eat at restaurants frequently,** eat as sensibly as you would at home. An everyday restaurant meal should not be treated as a special event.

☞ **Ask how various dishes are prepared.**

☞ Think "no cream, no cheese, no butter."

☞ **Scan the menu** and avoid dishes that have "cream" in the name or description, or that say "pan-fried," "crispy," "au gratin," or "scalloped."

☞ **Order foods broiled or grilled rather than fried.**

☞ **Order vegetables steamed, without butter added.**

☞ **Ask that sauces and salad dressings be served on the side.**

☞ Beware of fat- and oil-laden dishes at the salad bar.

☞ **Avoid rich, creamy desserts.** Opt instead for fresh fruit, sorbet, or fruit pie (and go easy on the crust).

☞ **Eat something at home before going out to a dinner party.**

Chapter Nine
Strategies for Eating In

Strategies

for

Eating In

"When Mama Got 'The Consciousness'"
– Deborah Levy

The year was 1988. Well, actually it was 1987, but it wasn't until '88 that we realized what had happened. Daddy was on a special low-fat diet for his heart, and Mama had sacrificed good cooking of her own free will. She devoted her kitchen time to making cardboard taste good. Though it was Daddy who was on the diet, it was Mama who became a fanatic. When she got The Consciousness, no one was safe. Not only family members, but friends, acquaintances, and people at neighboring tables in restaurants got the benefit of her wisdom. Up and down the East Coast, Mama preached the evils of red meat, heavy cream, and egg yolks.

None of us realized just how far she had gone until June, when we gave a cocktail party. As my brother and I were making a list of things to get (cheese and crackers, nuts) Mama looked at us as if we'd gone insane. "Nobody eats that stuff anymore," she informed us. It was evident that she felt we had failed her. But she valiantly took our education in hand and explained the need for celery, carrots, and a dip made from nonfat yogurt. My brother and I looked at each other in despair.

How To Cope With Family Rebellion

Just try to do something that's good for your family, and they'll turn against you every time, particularly when it involves a change of eating habits. Too bad, because while it's well and good to go out to dinner once in a while (Well and good? It's the best), more often than not you'll find yourself eating at home with the family.

Eating in. The opposite of eating out, in more ways than one, especially if you're in charge of meal planning, shopping, preparation, and cleanup.

Eating in may well involve other family members, small family mem-

Strategies

for

Eating In

bers, kids. As it happens, one of the things that makes kids what they are is their resistance to change, at least when it has to do with the way things have always been done at home. Many's the child who greeted Mother's new hairdo with "Yuk! I liked the old way better!" and other equally endearing remarks. Or reacted with dismay upon discovering a new brand of dishwashing liquid on the counter, not that the child ever washes the dishes, mind you.

It comes as no surprise to hear that a great many youngsters are not what you'd call interested in trying new things to eat. You may have to introduce a child to a new food as many as *fourteen times* before it is familiar enough to really eat, not just pick at.[24] Children vastly prefer foods that are instantly recognizable, not to mention overwhelmingly familiar, in both appearance and taste. Their idea of gourmet runs to the sorts of things that sponsor Saturday morning cartoon shows.

Now that a new day is dawning for you in the area of food preparation, you're undoubtedly aware that Junior may not take kindly to the requisite changes. Perhaps you can already envision the dinner table conversation:

"Ugh! What's this?"

"How can you say 'Ugh' when you haven't even taken a bite yet?"

"And I'm not taking a bite, either. No way! I want fried chicken!"

Be grateful if that's Junior talking, not your spouse.

The Jack Sprat Award for Low-Fat Products

Remember that you are not alone in this effort, because there are an enormous number of products on the market that can help you in your shift to low-fat cooking, more products all the time, and a few of them deserve special mention. They were available at a time when it was not so easy to locate low-fat products, and, while others have followed suit, these seem to us to have been Leaders of the Pack. Now, while a number of fat-

Strategies

for

Eating In

free foods have a taste level roughly akin to the cover of this book, these products **DO NOT**. Besides tasting very good, they: ❶ contain no added fat; ❷ are convenient. (Some also contain a lot of sodium,[25] and if that's something you specifically have to watch out for, then watch out here.)

With gratitude and appreciation,
we present the
Jack Sprat Award for Low-Fat Excellence to:
College Inn Chicken Broth (Lower Salt)
Contadina Light Garden Vegetable Sauce (for pasta)
Fleischmann's egg beaters
Health Valley Fat-Free Soups
Fantastic Foods, Knorr, and Nile Spice dehydrated soups
Near East Barley Pilaf, Lentil Pilaf, Spanish Rice
Pritikin Soups
Swanson Clear Vegetable Broth
Yves Veggie Wieners

We offer a sub-category of the Jack Sprat Award,
products that are low sodium as well as low fat:
Eden canned beans
Eden canned crushed tomatoes, "no salt added"
Fantastic Foods "Only a Pinch" dehydrated soups
Health Valley chicken broth, "no salt added"
Hunt's Tomato Sauce, "no salt added"

◆   ◆   ◆   ◆

Even with this kind of help, you may harbor fears about slaving over a hot stove only to have noses turn up at the dishes you've prepared. You may picture yourself lecturing about children who go to bed hungry every night, even as you are dimly aware that this tactic is hardly designed to win anybody over. But what *is* the best way to win them over?

How To Make Changes That Will Win Your Family's Heart

Strategies

for

Eating In

For one thing, don't make a big deal about all of this. There's no need to give a major address on the subject of eating healthfully, ending with something like, "You can bet your boots there are going to be some changes around here, folks!" Such an approach is guaranteed to draw the battle lines, which you'd clearly rather not do. Milk is a good place to begin quietly reducing fat in the family diet. If the family is used to drinking whole milk, switch first to 2 percent fat, then to 1 percent and finally to skim. We know, we know. Compared to whole milk, skim tastes watery. But once the family is used to 1 percent, skim won't taste much different. **(Note: Discuss any changes in diet with your pediatrician. Young children should not reduce fat the way older people should.)** Two percent-fat milk sounds really low in fat, but the truth is that the "2 percent fat" refers to weight, not calories. (Remember the "97% fat free" lunch meat that was really closer to 50% fat, discussed on page 40? Same principle applies here.) That is, when you drink a glass of this particular milk, 35 percent of the calories you are consuming come from fat. About 50 percent of the calories in whole milk come from fat. Truly "low-fat" milk is not the 2 percent-fat variety, even though the container says it is. One percent-fat milk does qualify as low fat, delivering 23 percent of its calories as fat; skim milk delivers virtually no fat at all.

You can introduce new foods gradually, too. Don't suddenly present things so wildly different from the usual fare that those gathered around the dinner table will wonder if this is their house. You might want to make some of the "embarrassingly simple" recipes in this book (beginning on page 131), and start by serving them along with other dishes that your family eats all the time. As you move farther away from the familiar, bring in reinforcements, serving plenty of pasta or rice or potatoes, plenty of fresh vegetables, and a good loaf of bread.

Milk is a good place to begin quietly reducing fat in the family diet.

Strategies

for

Eating In

Chicken, the Transition Food

We are a chicken-eating country. That's good, because, unless the chicken is fried (sorry, Junior), it's a low-fat choice. Even people who are not trying to eat a healthier diet are accidentally doing just that when they eat baked or broiled chicken.

Even though it's better to eat chicken than a different part of the cow every night, eating a lot of chicken is not a goal, not an end in itself. It is not The Ideal Entrée because there is no such thing, variety being the key.

But because chicken has broad-based appeal, can be prepared in so many ways, and is low in fat, it may be seen as a kind of "transition food," with the ability to move Americans in the direction of healthier eating.

By the way, have you noticed that Kentucky Fried Chicken is taking advantage of chicken's link with good health, and now calls itself KFC? Are we supposed to forget what that stands for? If the Colonel had made his fortune touting Kentucky Broiled Chicken, you can bet your drumstick they wouldn't be using initials today.

Chicken: Recipe Ideas

Rather than turn you loose and back to KFC–call it what you will, it's fried, folks – we offer (in addition to the "embarrassingly simple" chicken recipes beginning on page 136) several fast, easy, low-fat chicken recipe ideas. Note that these are only ideas, around which you can build your own recipes if you wish. Use skinless chicken.

Snow
Chicken

▼

■ Marinate breasts in fat-free bottled dressing, to which you've added chopped onion and garlic. Cook on the grill. The grill, by the way, can be used all year round. Never use it indoors, though, because it gives off noxious fumes. If there's snow on the ground, no problem. If there's snow on the grill, brush it off. Grilled food is delicious – "Snow Chicken" – and you can get away with using a lot less fat. (Don't blacken the food, though, because charred food is not particularly good for you to eat.)

■ Cut chicken into strips before marinating and cooking on the grill. (Or use chicken "tenders," small pieces of chicken breast that you'll find in the supermarket with the other poultry.) Add to pasta. You might also sauté zucchini in a tiny bit of olive oil (1 teaspoon per serving, tops) and add that, too. Finish with a good tomato sauce.

■ Cut up uncooked chicken and stir-fry with vegetables in a bit of oil (1 teaspoon per serving, tops). A little chicken goes a long way.

■ Poach chicken in a small amount of chicken broth. Add onion, carrot, and celery (without the chicken skin, you'll need some help to create flavor). By the way, if you are using canned broth, store it in the refrigerator. Why clutter up your already crowded refrigerator with canned broth? Because fat congeals on the top of the refrigerated broth, and you can just scrape off the fat and have fat-free broth.

■ After the above chicken is poached, remove vegetables and purée them in a food processor to serve with the chicken. Season to taste, and serve over rice or couscous (little pasta bits that kids love).

A Typical Meal
Meatballs

Low-fat meals need not feature chicken, of course. Even in the most extreme fat-consuming households, the change can

> ### DON'T FORGET ABOUT TURKEY
> A couple of hints:
> ■ There's no need to wait until Thanksgiving to serve turkey. Every once in a while cook a fresh turkey breast, lower in fat than the rest of the turkey, and much easier to prepare (either roast it or see recipe for Grilled Turkey Breast, page 142).
> ■ If you decide to use ground turkey as a replacement for hamburger, be sure to buy ground turkey *breast*. If you don't, you'll be eating meat that has skin ground up in it, and the result will be not only fatty but pretty gruesome to contemplate.

be easy and subtle. The trick is to start with the most acceptable dish (from the standpoint of this new way of eating) that has been served routinely, and go from there.

Say that the most acceptable dish is spaghetti and meatballs made with an old family recipe for tomato sauce. (Let's hope you're not dousing it with old-fashioned grated cheese.) First, the meatballs. Are you using the very leanest ("Extra Lean") ground beef you can buy? You can fur-

Use "Extra Lean" ground beef in your meatballs.

ther reduce fat by replacing some of the ground meat with bread crumbs.

When you cook the meatballs, do you sort of fry them in their own fat? If you do, instead try making tiny patties and putting them under the broiler so that the fat will run off. (Remember to turn them so they will brown on both sides.)

Sauce

Now the sauce. What's in that "old family recipe"? (In case your old family didn't make pasta sauce, or if you'd rather not bother, there are a number of no-added-fat choices on the market. Some are in jars. Contadina Light Garden Vegetable Sauce is very good and is refrigerated.)

If you do make your own sauce and the only fat is a little olive oil, you're all right. (Remember, one teaspoon per serving.) But if the recipe includes pork fat and other unacceptable ingredients, work on adapting the recipe. Anyone who makes tomato sauce from scratch is not a rank amateur as far as cooking is concerned, so you're sure to be clever enough and inventive enough to re-work the fat content of the dish. You may want to add more mushrooms, onions, garlic, or herbs to replace the flavor that is lost when you take out the fat.

Bread

Do you serve garlic bread with this meal? If you buy it frozen, check the label. You'll be amazed at how much fat it has. If you make it yourself, don't bother. You're better off serving a nice hot, crusty loaf of bread, and it's especially good for sopping up that tomato sauce everybody's so crazy about.

Salad

It's likely that a salad accompanies this particular meal. A word about their dressings.

Salads live and die by their dressings. When delicately coated, the greens are supreme; when covered, they are overpowered. You'll know which way you fix your salads by what's left in the bowl when the salad is gone. If there is a puddle of dressing sitting in the bottom, then you

If there is a puddle of dressing sitting in the bottom, then you like your salad well soaked. Consider using one of the many fat-free versions now available.

like your salad well soaked. Consider using one of the many fat-free versions now available, although odds are you won't be absolutely crazy about the taste or the smell or the appearance. These dressings do, however, serve the purpose. And they make terrific marinades.

If the empty salad bowl is almost dry or is glistening, you obviously don't use a lot of dressing, preferring to taste the salad as well as the dressing. You might be surprised when we suggest that the best way to do that is to use a regular dressing – not reduced fat, not fat free. It tastes wonderful, smells wonderful, looks wonderful – and contains more fat per serving than we've been recommending. We feel that's a small price to pay if it means you are eating vegetable-filled salads.

You have two embarrassingly simple options when it comes to delicious dressings: homemade (See box) and ready-made.

Ready-made: Shake bottle, unscrew cap, and pour.

> ### OUR FAVORITE HOMEMADE:
> Put 1/4 cup olive oil, 1/8 cup red wine or balsamic vinegar, and 1 teaspoon Dijon mustard in a small jar. Shake well. That's it. Enough for a salad for four.

Dessert

When it comes to dessert, change is more difficult, and you'll meet with opposition if your family's idea of dessert has meant a sweet treat at the end of every meal.

One change involves making the sweet an occasional treat. Another involves checking the Dessert section of this book (beginning on page 178) and finding a low-fat sweet.

Yet another change involves choosing other sorts of desserts. Try to stick to fruit – fresh, dried, even canned (in its own juice rather than in heavy syrup). Summertime offers wonderful fresh fruits such as melons and berries, which combine to make a delicious fruit bowl. In winter, oranges and grapefruit can be sectioned. For company, put the sections with their juice in a bowl, add some cut-up strawberries, and mix in a bit of orange-flavored liqueur. You can put A Great Raspberry Sauce over the fruit, too (see recipe, page 181).

Strategies

for

Eating In

If you want to serve something baked, best of all is angel food cake, which contains no fat. You can serve it with fruit, or you can slice the cake in half, crosswise, and spread fruit topping between the layers. Or add unsweetened cocoa powder during baking, resulting in chocolate flavor without the fat found in chocolate (see recipe for "Chocolate" Angel Food Cake, page 187).

Presentation

As you think about new ways of preparing food, think, too, about the way it looks on the plate.

Imagine on your white dinner plate: a piece of poached flounder flanked by a baked potato and a helping of mashed turnips, with perhaps a crusty piece of bread on the side. Sounds like a healthy, low-fat meal, which is what we've been discussing this whole time, haven't we, for heaven's sake? Ah, but think about how the dinner looks. It may remind you of the picture you "drew" when you were a kid, a blank sheet of paper that you said was a polar bear in a snowstorm. Well, in fact the flounder/potato/turnip/bread might be just as hard to locate on that white dinner plate. It may taste good, but you start off with a couple of strikes against you in the presentation department.

In other words, you aren't taking advantage of the possibilities of advertising the meal you've just prepared. Short of investing in colored plates, admittedly a possible, if extravagant, solution, you'll want to begin to consider: ❶color; ❷texture; ❸garnish; and ❹arrangement of food.

An attractive plate of food contains a variety of colors. There is almost always something in the pink/red/orange/yellow group (salmon? red beets? red beans? tomatoes? sweet potatoes? carrots?); something in the green group (spinach? broccoli? asparagus? green beans? lima beans? artichoke? peas?); and something in the white or brown group (pasta? rice? potato? meat? chicken? fish?).

> **HOT TIP:**
>
> You won't stick to this new way of eating for the rest of your life if the food doesn't look appealing and appetizing.

Variety in texture is also pleasant, which is why you probably wouldn't serve mashed potatoes and mashed carrots at the same meal, unless you were trying out some new piece of kitchen equipment and got carried away.

Contrary to popular opinion, restaurants don't have the exclusive right to garnish a dinner plate. Maybe you don't want to bother with rosettes and things, but try steaming some carrot "coins" or slivered carrots just to put on the plate to add some color. You can do the same with purple cabbage. If you're in a hurry (and who isn't?), don't even bother cooking them first. They'll still add the color and serve the purpose. You can eat them uncooked, too.

Finally, the way you arrange food on the plate can enhance both the appearance of the food and the pleasure of eating it, so take a few seconds to make things look attractive.

There is definitely more to eating than putting food in your mouth. Interestingly, the Japanese consider all of this so important that their country's dietary guidelines state that experiences related to eating must be pleasurable. And if you fill all the senses, you'll be less likely to overcompensate in one: taste.

How To Be A Smart Shopper

When you eat in, you shop out. Often. Each week, you might go to the supermarket one day (or two or three or four days), to a farm stand another day, and maybe to a convenience store yet another day, to pick up something you've run out of or forgotten to buy on a previous trip. And now, with your new-found interest in healthy eating, you'll be looking for what you consider to be healthy foods. For example, you may decide to add health food stores to your already long list of places to grocery shop, since they are known for carrying additive- and preservative-free foods. And they do, after all, have the word "health" in their name.

*"Natural"
doesn't
necessarily
mean the
food is low
in fat.*

If you've never done so, walk into one sometime. You'll find starches in the form of unusual dried beans, whole grains, flours. You'll find platters of enormous, all-natural muffins, and breads with the whole grains bursting forth. You'll find containers of nuts and seeds and granola; "meats" made from soybeans. (Meats aren't alone in their soybean connection: Henry Ford envisioned using soybean plastics to build cars.)[26] You'll find magazines printed on recycled paper, cookbooks with names like *The Whole Grain Cookbook* and *Cooking with Nuts*, and cosmetics that haven't been tested on animals. When you reach the check-out counter at a health food store, they never ask if you want "paper or plastic." They often ask if you want a bag at all, figuring you may very well have brought along your own, as so many of their environmentally conscious customers do. If you do need a bag, the one you'll get may very well be creased and worn.

What with the shelves filled with boxes and bags and jars of foods made by companies that don't advertise on television, and that feature the words "ORGANIC" and "NATURAL INGREDIENTS," you have the feeling that you could close your eyes and fill your cart, and, no matter what you took home, you'd be in good shape.

But you have to remember that, whether in a supermarket or a health food store or anywhere else, you must be an intelligent consumer. "Natural" doesn't necessarily mean the food is low in fat.

Take granola, for example. There it is, maybe in a barrel the size of a three-year-old child, a barrel with a big metal scoop lying on top. Somewhere in the vicinity is a hand-lettered sign that says "GRANOLA" executed in calligraphy. The name itself has an aura of healthy living, and granola even looks healthy, with its fully formed steel cut flakes of oats, its generous amounts of nuts, and its natural sweeteners in the form of raisins and dates. It's a complete meal in a bowl: fruit (raisins and dates), starch (oats), and protein (nuts).

Don't Forget About Fat

But the big question is, as is the case with all the foods you buy, wherever you buy them: How much fat are you getting? Unless this is a fat-free granola, chances are you are getting a fair amount. How do you know? By looking at the granola and seeing nuts, which tips you off to the fact that this is a food higher in fat, and by reading the label, which will be on or near the bulk container.

If it isn't reduced fat or fat free, granola (wherever you buy it) contains somewhere in the neighborhood of 1 teaspoon of fat (5 grams) in 1/4 cup. But think about that serving size. One-quarter cup is a garnish, not a serving. A normal breakfast helping might be closer to one cup (think OPSS – Own Personal Serving Size), which would be 20 grams of fat, or 4 teaspoons. On top of that, maybe you grab snacks throughout the day. How many grams in a fistful? Who knows? Depends on the size of your hand. YOU MUST BE AWARE OF SERVING SIZE, WHEREVER YOU BUY YOUR FOOD. IT HAS EVERYTHING TO DO WITH THE AMOUNT OF FAT YOU TAKE IN.

Reminder: No matter where you buy your food, pay attention to serving size.

Label Free May Not Be Fat Free

When you select foods without standard labeling, you move into the realm of the unknown. Take those muffins mentioned earlier. They are the size of headlight bulbs. They are lumpy, oddly-shaped, and look, in a word, homemade. The question is, how much fat will you be getting if you take one home? Or eat it in the car? Or on your way to the car? Since by law labels do not have to appear on foods prepared on the premises, or by small businesses, you have no way of knowing the fat content. Maybe someone at the store can help you, or, if you're lucky, there will be a "fat free" sign next to the muffins. (If there is no sign, you might try the old "napkin test," which involves setting a muffin on a paper napkin, then taking it off and looking for a telltale grease spot. Too bad that, by the time you see the spot, you are already the proud owner of a fat-laden muffin.)

Often the packaging in health food stores is alluring because the

Strategies

for

Eating In

approach is different. It's the softest of soft sells, but it's a sell nonetheless. The companies whose products inhabit the shelves of health food stores have names such as Fantastic Foods, Erewhon, Tree of Life, Love Natural Foods, Nature's Choice, and After the Fall. Just remember that these are companies exactly like Beatrice, Kraft, General Mills, or Nabisco, and that their goal is to sell their products. And just because the names suggest happiness, peace of mind, and well-being, you must, repeat must, read labels in order to find out whether or not a given product is low in fat.

Moving On

I t's a lot easier to talk about eating low fat than it is to maintain a low-fat way of eating. Sometimes it seems as if everything is against you. In fact, when we were writing an early draft of this book on the computer, merrily cutting and pasting away, the computer merged two sections accidentally, and the following sentences came out of the printer. This is true, really. We swear it. Besides, who could make up something like this?

> If you are feeling creative, ask the butcher to take the bone out and the skin off of a turkey breast. When you get home and take it out of the package, it won't look wildly appetizing, but don't despair. Rinse it in cold water, pat dry with paper towels, then cut some slashes in it and put it in a roasting pan. *Stick some cloves of garlic in the slashes, dump a little lemon juice in there, too, and rub the whole thing with pork fat and other unacceptable ingredients* [italics added].

So here you are, providing nutritious and, you hope, delicious meals for your family, meeting with occasional resistance nevertheless ("How come we never have fried chicken anymore?"). But if you are determinedly upbeat, secure in the knowledge that you are preparing healthful, tasty meals, chances are good that they'll come around eventually. Teens might do so more readily if some smart rock group would call itself "Low Fat," so that the word would get out via T-shirts, but in the meantime you'll have to do the best you can.

Speaking of teenagers, you might well wonder how you can control what they eat outside the house. It's one thing to stock the refrigerator and cupboard with the "right" foods, but how about when they're out with their friends (read "at the mall")? Well, the simple fact is that some things are out of your control, and this is one of them. Still, just as basic values are instilled at home and are then put into practice by kids out in the big, wide world, this, too, will be an effort you will make at home and hope that some of it rubs off for more permanent use elsewhere. Besides, what you serve at home will help balance the high-fat choices they make on their own, and the daily total of fat consumption will therefore average out more favorably.

Take comfort in the fact that all improvements you make put family members that much ahead of the game, whatever they do on their own. You don't want to be in the position of monitoring everyone's food intake, which would be not only incredibly boring, but also nonproductive in a number of ways, not the least of which would be enormous family friction. There's just so much you yourself can do.

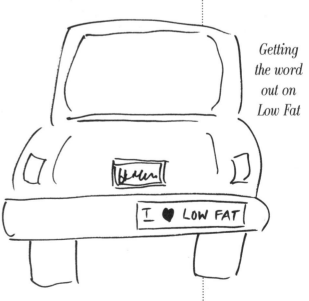

*Getting
the word
out on
Low Fat*

Chapter 9

Strategies

for

Eating In

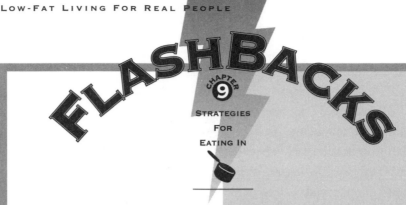

FLASHBACKS

CHAPTER 9
STRATEGIES
FOR
EATING IN

☞ **Introduce changes gradually:**
- Offer skim or 1 percent-fat milk.
- Reduce fat in dishes you normally prepare.
- Serve an "embarrassingly simple" dish, along with the usual fare.

☞ **It's okay – a good idea, even – to serve more than one starch and vegetable per meal.**

☞ **Grill, broil, or poach rather than fry.**

☞ **Reduce serving sizes of protein foods** (meat/poultry/fish/cheese).

☞ **Read food labels wherever you shop,** including health food stores.

☞ **Make sure the food you serve looks attractive** and colorful, and that it offers a variety of textures.

☞ **Relax** and accept that you cannot control what family members eat on their own time.

☞ **Remember** – you can only do what you can do.

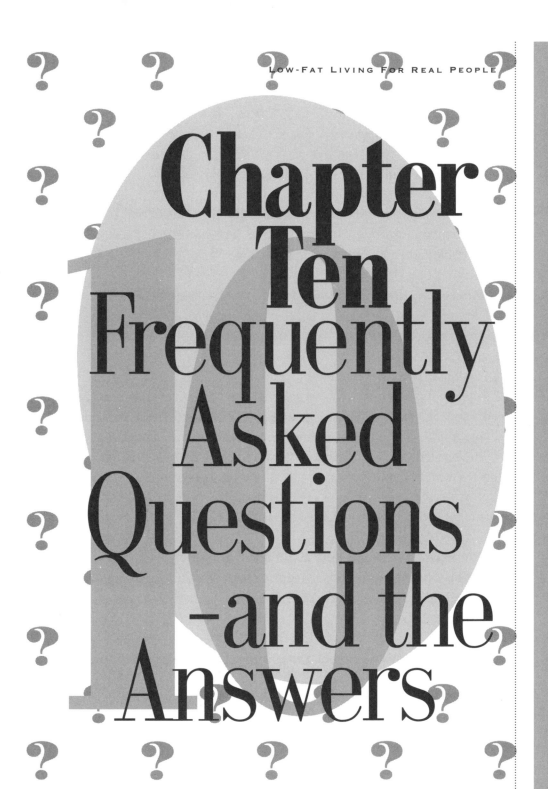

Chapter Ten
Frequently Asked Questions – and the Answers

CHAPTER
10

Frequently

Asked

Questions

– and the

Answers

?

Frequently

Asked

Questions

– and the

Answers

If these questions speak to you, you have a lot of company. They are questions that we've been asked (professionally and nonprofessionally) over and over again.

Q: Am I eating low fat if I buy only foods that say "Low Cholesterol"?

A: Not necessarily. You have to check the food label for total fat. Low cholesterol and low fat are not the same thing.[27]

Q: Am I eating low cholesterol if I eat foods that are low in fat?

A: Most likely. Foods that are low in fat tend to be low in cholesterol, with the exception of organ meats (brains, liver, kidneys).

Q: Isn't margarine better than butter?

A: No, it isn't, unless you've selected one of the new, nonhydrogenated versions (such as Nucoa Smart Beat), and even so, all the calories come from fat. The point to remember is that hydrogenated and partially hydrogenated fats are a definite "fats no-no." You absolutely, positively, do not want them in your diet. In the famous on-going Nurses' Health Study, nurses who consumed hydrogenated fat had more heart disease than those who did not consume the fat.

Q: If margarine is so bad, how about diet margarine?

A: Diet margarine is simply regular margarine with air beaten into it, meaning there is less fat in a serving. Still, when you're not eating air, you're eating fat.

Q: Not to push this margarine thing, but what am I supposed to use on my toast in the morning?

A: Try jam, jelly, marmalade, honey. They contain no fat at all.

Q: Are you suggesting that I fry with jam or jelly?

A: No, we're suggesting that you don't fry at all! Nonstick skillets are wonderful, and if you still need a bit of fat, use spray oil, which you can get in the supermarket. But use it sparingly.

Q: What about the new fat-free mayonnaise, cream cheese, sour cream, and all that?

A: When you decide to go easy on fat, this is a great way to begin, assuming you don't mind the loss of taste (less apparent when you are combining a number of ingredients in a recipe). And these products offer the comfort of the familiar without the fat. However, there are new and wonderful tastes out there, tastes that go beyond the creaminess of mayonnaise and sour cream, and you'll want to try them. Check out the recipes in the back of this book.

Q: In order to eat "low fat," do I have to eat vegetarian?

A: No, no, no, no, no! Absolutely not!

Still, if only for the sake of variety, it's kind of nice to eat vegetarian every once in a while (pasta's always good), but remember that vegetarian dishes are not necessarily low in fat. Again, the recipes in the back of this book will give you lots of ideas.

Q: I've heard that bananas are fatty. Is that true?

A: No. Bananas don't contain fat. Fruits, as well as vegetables, are as close as you can get to no-fat foods. There are a few fatty exceptions, such as avocados and olives, and you simply have to go easy on these.

As far as gaining weight goes, you'd have to eat an awful lot of bananas to gain weight. How many overweight monkeys have you seen lately?

Q: What do I do about salt on a low-fat diet?

A: Naturally your body is happier without too much salt, but low-fat eating is a separate issue. In other words, you don't have to eat less salt on a low-fat diet.

Q: How about sugar? If I eat low sugar, will I be eating low fat?

A: Probably not. While it's true that lots of sugary foods also contain a whole lot of fat (ice cream, baked goods, et cetera), sugar and fat are not the same thing. Eating less sugar doesn't mean you are also eating

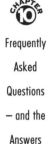

Frequently
Asked
Questions
– and the
Answers

less fat. Besides, if you eat many sugary foods, you won't be eating all the "good stuff" (okay, okay, we all have our own definition of "good stuff") like fruits and vegetables, which really are low in fat.

Q: Can't I just take a vitamin instead of lowering the fat in my diet?

A: There is no substitute for a low-fat diet. Vitamins can't make fat go away. Maybe you've heard people say, "I wish there was a magic pill for this." We all do. And we're still looking for one.

Q: What about these fat-free cakes and cookies I keep hearing about?

A: Ah, you mean Fat-Free Chocolate-Covered Creme-Filled Mini-Cakes. They are popular, all right, and we suppose they're an option if eaten occasionally and in intelligent serving sizes. They have no nutritional value, though. And they have plenty of calories. Fat free doesn't mean calorie free.

Q: I'm sick and tired of chicken! Is there anything else I can eat instead?

A: Sounds like you're in a "chicken rut." Food is like a theme park. Obviously you don't always want to take the same ride. So try other rides! See the next question.

Q: Can I eat beef? Pork?

A: Yes, but not all the time, maybe once or twice a week. Check labels for "Extra Lean" or "Lean," preferably the former, which is lower in fat. Remember to think "deck of cards," not "placemat," when it comes to serving size.

Q: Can I eat shrimp?

A: Yes, and ignore those who make comments about the cholesterol it contains. Again, don't eat it all the time, and pay attention to that 3-ounce serving size. If you buy 6 ounces of raw shrimp in the shell, you will have 3 ounces of cooked shrimp at home.[28]

Q: Should I avoid fatty fish?

A: No. All fish is good for you, and the fat in fish is not the kind of fat you have to worry about.

Q: I hate this. How about if I just eat "Healthy Choice" for lunch and dinner every day?

A: You're going to get very, very bored. After a while everything will begin to taste the same, and you'll get sick of the whole thing and give up even the pretense of eating low fat. The trick is to commit yourself to finding new foods that taste good and are easy to prepare. Which is, after all, one reason why you bought this book, isn't it?

Q: I like to eat pizza on Friday nights. Any suggestions?

A: We assume you want to continue this tradition, so why not make the pizza as low in fat as possible? While you're at it, go out with like-minded friends so you can order one pizza with extra vegetables instead of the usual (high in fat) pepperoni or sausage. Then ask for half the cheese. In fact, many places now make delicious no-cheese pizzas. Finally, have a salad and extra bread so two slices will satisfy you.

Q: It's holiday time! I look forward to this all year! Are you suggesting that I give up my traditional holiday treats?

A: Of course not. Eat and enjoy. We are, however, suggesting that you not *over*eat. When you really, truly binge, you feel really, truly terrible anyway, and there you are popping antacid tablets (admittedly fat free). But if you just go easy, even though you may be eating high-fat foods, you won't be eating so much of them, which will automatically mean lower fat. Also, you might want to introduce one low-fat dish to the holiday table – maybe Pumpkin Pie-less, a pumpkin custard (see recipe, page 186).

Q: What if I crave chocolate, which I know is high in fat?

A: Go for fat free! Use Hershey's syrup. Eat a fat-free Fudgsicle. Have a cup of Alba hot cocoa. Or get yourself a small chocolate bar, preferably dark chocolate, which appears to be less damaging to the heart. Better than buying the extraordinarily large, pass-around size that you'll eat all by yourself anyhow. By the way, if you buy the most expensive chocolate bar you can find, you'll be less likely to get the large size.

Q: I love good ice cream. I've tried that nonfat frozen yogurt, but it's a pretty bad substitute. Any ideas?

A: Check out various brands of nonfat frozen yogurt. Some are, we admit, not much in the flavor department, but others are very good. Taste being the individual issue that it is, you'll want to "taste test" for yourself. If all else fails, you're better off with a small amount of low-fat frozen yogurt rather than going back to premium ice cream. If you are buying a cup of frozen yogurt at the mall, say, Colombo's is a good nonfat choice. If you are standing in the freezer section at the supermarket, remember to read labels. Many frozen yogurts are quite high in fat. Breyer's is an example of one that is low in fat; Dannon and Sealtest Free are nonfat.

Q: I've checked the Ingredient List on my bread and pasta, just like you want me to do, and I see that there is no added fat. So how come the Nutrition Facts label tells me there is 1 gram of fat?

A: Small amounts of fat occur naturally in grains. Don't worry about it.

Q: My kids and my spouse eat low fat at home, but as soon as they leave the house, it's another story. What can I do about that?

A: Not much. You have obviously set an example at home, and that's about all you can do.

Q: My spouse will not eat low fat. What can I do about *that*?

A: We assume you're doing the cooking, which means that you are probably not cooking the same way you used to. You might try making some of the old favorites from time to time, and negotiating the rest.

And give yourself time – months, maybe many months. This doesn't have to happen overnight. Remember that anything you can do to reduce fat in the diet is helpful, and that even the smallest step is a step in the right direction.

Frequently

Asked

Questions

– and the

Answers

Chapter Eleven

How to Use Food Labels to Select Low-Fat Foods

How to Use

Food Labels

to Select

Low-Fat Foods

Anti-Dedication

*To the Food and Drug Administration, for coming up with
the all but unintelligible term "Daily Value"
and making the label chapter of this book so hard to write*

Understanding the Food Label

We've been talking a lot about choosing foods that are low in fat – the kinds of meats, the kinds of starches, the kinds of snacks that fit into a low-fat diet. We've seen that what you assume to be low in fat may not be (think of SMART-FOOD popcorn). Then, too, misleading claims made in advertisements (on television and in magazines, for instance)[29] greatly complicate the task of people everywhere who are knocking themselves senseless trying to avoid fat.

Now labels give you a shot at figuring out how much fat is in the foods you buy, because, after years of controversy, new, non-deceiving labels have come to the packages of food in your supermarket. Well, not to all packages. If they are too small, like Vienna sausages, or the companies are too small, like Uncle John's Magic Morning Tofu Drink, or if the food is a raw food,[30] or is located in the bakery or the delicatessen section, it doesn't have to have a label. If the food in question happens to be raw meat or poultry, it doesn't have to have a label either. Too bad, because there's plenty of fat in there. Add all this to the fact that no nutrition information is required on the breads, rolls, and cakes, the freshly sliced lunch meats and cheeses, the prepared salads and appetizers, the desserts – well, let's just say they aren't making things easy for us, are they? Check the Endnote[31] for specific information on fat content. Be prepared to have your socks knocked off.

The food labels are clear and easy to look at, but the question is: Are they easy to understand? You have a fighting chance of understanding them if you pore over 1,000 pages of newsprint in the Federal Register.

And what exactly is the Federal Register? It's as if a secretary took notes at a meeting, only this meeting lasted for years and years, and on January 6, 1993, the notes were printed – in two volumes. This chapter will help you decide whether or not it was worth it.

How to Use
Food Labels
to Select
Low-Fat Foods

Take a look at the label. Looks like a math test, doesn't it? You might even feel that long ago, almost forgotten sensation of fear gripping your heart when you suddenly realized *you studied the wrong thing*! Now take a deep breath, and you'll realize something else: You are a victim of information overload. There is too much going on here, too much to take in.

The first words you see, in bold type, are Nutrition Facts (not what you'd call snappy). What follows are facts, all right, more than you could possibly be interested in, thirty-nine different facts on an average label, to be precise (yes, we counted), fat facts included, plus assorted typefaces and a variety of lines of different thicknesses, all packed into just a few square inches.

Nutrition Facts
Serving Size 1 cup (228g)
Servings Per Container 2

Amount Per Serving

Calories 260   Calories from Fat 120

	% Daily Value*
Total Fat 13g	**20%**
Saturated Fat 5g	**25%**
Cholesterol 30mg	**10%**
Sodium 660mg	**28%**
Total Carbohydrate 31g	**10%**
Dietary Fiber 0g	**0%**
Sugars 5g	
Protein 5g	

Vitamin A 4% • Vitamin C 2%

Calcium 15% • Iron 4%

* Percent Daily Values are based on a 2,000 calorie diet. Your daily values may be higher or lower depending on your calorie needs.

	Calories:	2,000	2,500
Total Fat	Less than	65g	80g
Sat Fat	Less than	20g	25g
Cholesterol	Less than	300mg	300mg
Sodium	Less than	2,400mg	2,400mg
Total Carbohydrate		300g	375g
Dietary Fiber		25g	30g

Calories per gram:
Fat 9 • Carbohydrate 4 • Protein 4

of different thicknesses, all packed into just a few square inches.

◆   ◆   ◆   ◆

Everyone agrees that most Americans should be reducing the amount of fat they take in.

Because there are so many facts, let's narrow our focus, and we'll bet you can guess that the focus will be, quite simply, on label information for fat. Calories from Fat. Total Fat. Saturated Fat.

All are given top billing. The label even tells you how the fat in the food relates to the other foods you eat that day. It's a clear statement that fat information is important, an emphasis that is mighty convenient for our purposes. Debates on proper eating rage all around us, but, as Dr. Timothy Johnson pointed out on ABC's "Nightline," we must make no

How to Use

Food Labels

to Select

Low-Fat Foods

mistake, the debate is not about lowering fat in the diet; *everyone agrees that most Americans should be reducing the amount of fat they take in.*

Daily Value

As far as the food label is concerned, the new kid on the block is Daily Value. (And you thought Nutrition Facts was dull and dry.) Remember when the government used to give guidelines for vitamins and minerals? RDA? Or was it U.S. RDA? Whatever. Now it's giving guidelines for fat, among other things, and calling them Daily Values, DV for short. It has never before ventured this. It's new. It's innovative. It's a nuisance, but let's push on anyway.

◆   ◆   ◆   ◆

A certain number of a day's calories can come from fat, but not too many: your "Daily Value."

From the sound of it, you might think Daily Value is a subject taught in Sunday School, but no. Daily Value is one day's worth of a given nutrient. Take fat, for example. (Well, the whole idea is that you *don't* take fat, but you get the idea.) You should eat no more than a given amount of fat each day, and that amount is the Daily Value.

This isn't the first time we've discussed Daily Value, it's just that we didn't call it by that name. We've talked (a whole lot) about The Big Picture, about eating less fat, about how we don't want to eat enough fat for an entire day at one sitting, and we've said that if we eat too much fat there are health risks. As we've seen, it all comes down to this: A certain number of a day's calories can come from fat, but not too many, **no more than 30 percent of the total number of calories you take in each day.** Now we'll give that a name: your "Daily Value." Considering that the average American eats upwards of a 39 percent fat diet, 30 percent is a significant improvement. But some studies have shown that even 30 percent isn't low enough. A therapeutic reduced-fat diet may be closer to *10 percent fat* and has, in fact, been shown by Dr. Dean Ornish to reverse heart disease, that is, clear the arteries.[32] (This diet is not for everyone, however, and should not be followed without professional guidance.)

Before we get to the Daily Value for fat, we'd like to point out that the label has a disclaimer: "Your Daily Values may be higher or lower depending on your calorie needs."[33] Translation: If you consume fewer than 2,000 calories in a day, you should be eating less fat than the 2,000-calorie types. It then follows that your Daily Value for fat is lower than the one on the label. ("Great, just great," we hear you say. We know. We agree.)

At the bottom of the new food label you'll see Daily Value calculated for fat, and here it is: *less than 65 grams, if you are a 2,000-calorie a day type*.[34] Who needs 2,000 calories a day (which is really only a ballpark figure)? An active teenage female; a very active middle-aged business-woman who exercises strenuously; a sedentary, middle-aged businessman (life is so unfair). Most women do not need 2,000 calories a day. This means that, for them, a 30 per-cent-fat diet would be considerably less than 65 grams of fat, and probably closer to *50 grams of fat*. (If they are trying to lose weight, even 50 grams of fat is high.)

Nevertheless, let's try to get a handle on the 65 grams Daily Value for fat. Put it in perspective, and all that. Each of the things we've talked about – Elvis's red-eye gravy, and the margarine used at mealtimes that amounted to half a stick, and the thirteen homemade oatmeal cookies, and the six-ounce bag of chips, and the box of Wheat Thins (which, if you're going to eat the entire box at one time, should be called "Wheat *Fats*"), and the whole bag of SMARTFOOD popcorn – all of these are pretty close to containing 65 grams of fat, the Daily Value for an entire day in one fell swoop (if you are a 2,000-calorie type).

And if you aren't, well, too bad you can't go to the super-market and find your own, personalized labels on each box. Given that we are stuck with a "one size fits all" label, and that the Daily Value may not exactly be appropriate for any one of us, it can help us see the big fat picture.

Enough background. Let's walk through the label together.

How to Use

Food Labels

to Select

Low-Fat Foods

Nutrition Facts

Serving Size 1 cup (228g)
Servings Per Container 2

Amount Per Serving

Calories 260   Calories from Fat 120

	% Daily Value*
Total Fat 13g	**20%**
Saturated Fat 5g	**25%**
Cholesterol 30mg	**10%**
Sodium 660mg	**28%**
Total Carbohydrate 31g	**10%**
Dietary Fiber 0g	**0%**
Sugars 5g	
Protein 5g	

Vitamin A 4% • Vitamin C 2%

Calcium 15% • Iron 4%

* Percent Daily Values are based on a 2,000 calorie diet. Your daily values may be higher or lower depending on your calorie needs.

		Calories:	2,000	2,500
Total Fat	Less than		65g	80g
Sat Fat	Less than		20g	25g
Cholesterol	Less than		300mg	300mg
Sodium	Less than		2,400mg	2,400mg
Total Carbohydrate			300g	375g
Dietary Fiber			25g	30g

Calories per gram:
Fat 9 • Carbohydrate 4 • Protein 4

How to Use

Food Labels

to Select

Low-Fat Foods

Nutrition Facts

Serving Size 1 cup (228g)
Servings Per Container 2

Amount Per Serving

Calories 260   Calories from Fat 120

	% Daily Value*
Total Fat 13g	**20%**
Saturated Fat 5g	**25%**

Serving Size

At the top of the label is Serving Size, and the big news here is that serving sizes are: ❶ expressed in common household measurements; and ❷ no longer up to the manufacturer. Under the old labeling system, manufacturers could create teeny-weeny serving sizes so that the per-serving fat content, for instance, looked appealing. Land O' Lakes Butter listed a one *teaspoon* serving while other companies used one *tablespoon*, leading unwary consumers to think Land O' Lakes was lower in fat, when the serving size was simply one third that of its competitors. Soda cans routinely listed "Servings per Container – 2," presumably in order to cut the calories in half. Show us someone who shares a soda and we'll show you someone who has either been coerced into sharing it or doesn't really like soda.

No more is this sort of deception allowed. Instead, the Food and Drug Administration (FDA) has researched the issue of how much people eat of a given food at one time, and that's considered the serving size. (If you like jargon, try the FDA's definition of serving size: "An amount of food customarily consumed per eating occasion by persons 4 years of age or older which is expressed in a common household measure that is appropriate to the food.") Understand that this is the amount commonly consumed. It is not a *recommended* amount.

Besides, the serving sizes don't necessarily bear much resemblance to the amount you, personally, eat. As we've encouraged you to do throughout this book, *think OPSS (Own Personal Serving Size) when reading a label.* How big is your serving? Compare it to the amount on the label and you may find that you have some calculating to do. (Remember, it doesn't take much to go from OPSS to OOPS!) It makes no difference what the label calls "one serving"; if you eat two or three times that, then everything else on the label, grams of fat included, will have to be multiplied by two or three or whatever. *Serving Size is the most important item on the label, because everything that follows is based on that.*

Amount Per Serving:
Calories and Calories from Fat

Next you see, on a per-serving basis, how many calories are in the product and how many calories come from fat. These figures tell you at a glance how much fat is in the food. In this case, there are 260 calories per serving, 120 of which come from fat. Pretty high, don't you think? But the important thing, from the point of view of label reading, is the emphasis given to fat content.

Total Fat: Grams

As you look at this label, you can see that Nutrition Facts about fat are presented in two other ways as well. One, which has been around for a long time, simply gives the grams of fat in a serving of the food. (As we've seen earlier in this book, a gram is a unit of weight, about that of a straight pin.) You can consider that the product is low in fat if it contains no more than 3 grams of fat in one serving.

The other way in which fat information is presented is Percent Daily Value.

Nutrition Facts

Serving Size 1 cup (228g)
Servings Per Container 2

Amount Per Serving	
Calories 260 Calories from Fat 120	

	% Daily Value
Total Fat 13g	20%
Saturated Fat 5g	25%
Cholesterol 30mg	10%
Sodium 660mg	28%
Total Carbohydrate 31g	10%
Dietary Fiber 0g	0%
Sugars 5g	
Protein 5g	

Total Fat: Percent Daily Value

Now that you understand what Daily Value is – how many grams of fat, say, that you might reasonably eat in a day – we come to "*Percent Daily Value*." See it? Over on the right? "% Daily Value"? Ah, numbers, numbers, numbers.

Percent Daily Value for fat is the relationship between the amount of fat in a serving of that product and the total amount of fat you might reasonably eat in a day (Daily Value). Now this may (May? Did someone say *may*?) sound complicated and off-putting, and it is, really. But let's press on. We've almost got it.

Why the percentages? Because consumer studies found that people couldn't tell if 13 grams, for instance, was a lot of fat or a little fat, but if they were told it was 20 percent of a whole day's worth of fat (Daily

How to Use

Food Labels

to Select

Low-Fat Foods

Value), it was easier to understand. To repeat: Percent Daily Value will tell you what percentage of a day's fat is found in one serving of the food if you eat 2,000 calories a day, because, as we've seen over and over again, the Daily Values (and now Percent Daily Values) on every single label are based on a 2,000-calorie diet.

So what about these percentages? Who do these people think we are, anyway? Mathematicians? If you go to the supermarket with a calculator, chances are you intend to add up the prices, not figure out how much fat you're getting. Or worry about the fact that you may be trying to eat less than a 30 percent fat diet, but they've calculated 30 percent here, and, to make matters worse, you may be one of those people who doesn't need 2,000 calories a day.

Are the percentages useful if you consume more or less than 2,000 calories? Well, yes, sort of. You just can't take them too literally. The Percent Daily Value for fat can be used as a screening mechanism that tells you at a glance whether there's a lot or a little fat in the particular product, and therefore whether or not you should even consider buying it. So look for the foods that have:

5% OR LESS DAILY VALUE FOR TOTAL FAT [35]

Since you eat something like twenty different foods each day, you don't want to get most of your fat by eating just one or two of them, because you'll be way over your limit by lunchtime.

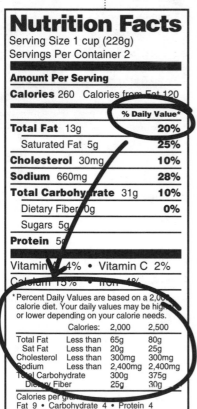

Everything You Never Wanted to Know About Daily Values

Follow the bouncing asterisk to the bottom of Nutrition Facts and you will see, in small print, other Daily Values. Do you care about them? Should you care about them? Of course you should. Saturated Fat and Cholesterol are biggies, but things are getting pretty complicated, so simplify matters by establishing priorities. You won't be surprised when we suggest that you rivet your attention on TOTAL FAT.

You'll also see Daily Values for Sodium, Total Carbohydrate, and Dietary Fiber (whoever names these things isn't exactly a stand-up comic), which do not contain fat. As you know by now, if you're filling up on pasta and beans (examples of Carbohydrate and Fiber), you'll be eating less fat.

Then you'll see information relating not only to a diet of 2,000 calories, which we've just discussed, but also for 2,500 calories. Why? Good question, since the percentages on the label are based on 2,000 calories, and this just becomes confusing. Too much information.

Saturated Fat

At the risk of causing motion sickness, we ask you to go back up the label, this time to Saturated Fat ("Sat Fat" to its friends, if it had any). The truth is, you should be eliminating it from your diet as much as you possibly can. This is not easy, particularly if you eat animal products (meat, poultry, cheese), since that's where most Saturated Fat is found. It's so incredibly undesirable that to be considered low Saturated Fat, a serving of food may contain no more than 1 gram of that fat. You might prefer to go with a more general screening device, and you'll see it's identical to the one we used for Total Fat:

5% OR LESS DAILY VALUE FOR SATURATED FAT

NOTE

Avoid Hydrogenated and Partially Hydrogenated Fat because they are "sat fat two-fers," containing both sat fat and *trans* fat. To repeat what we've said before, they are commonly found in margarine, in chips, in crackers, in cookies, and in other commercially baked goods. Since they are not (as of this writing) listed as such in Nutrition Facts, you'll have to check the Ingredient List to see if they are present.

Nutrition Facts

Serving Size 1 cup (228g)
Servings Per Container 2

Amount Per Serving

Calories 260　Calories from Fat 120

	% Daily Value*
Total Fat 18g	20%
Saturated Fat 5g	25%
Cholesterol 30mg	10%
Sodium 660mg	28%
Total Carbohydrate 31g	10%
Dietary Fiber 0g	0%

*A Useful
Guide:
5% OR
LESS DAILY
VALUE IS
LOW*

Cholesterol

As for Cholesterol: If your diet is low in Saturated Fat, it is low in Cholesterol (if you're not eating organ meats), so you don't have to worry about Daily Value for Cholesterol, which is, by the way, the same for all adults: less than 300 milligrams a day. A food is considered low in Cholesterol if it contains 20 milligrams or less per serving.

Percent Daily Value again becomes a useful guide when it comes to screening for Cholesterol – and there's that 5% again:

5% OR LESS DAILY VALUE FOR CHOLESTEROL

> ### IN A NUTSHELL
> Good old grams can still be used when selecting foods that are low in Total Fat, Saturated Fat, and Cholesterol, but you have to remember different amounts for each. However, a glance at Percent Daily Value will tell you if a food is low in Total Fat, Saturated Fat, and Cholesterol:
> **5% OR LESS IS LOW**

Sodium

Sodium, not really related to fat, has an unchanging Daily Value of 2,400 milligrams no matter how many calories you take in. A food qualifies as "low sodium" if it contains 140 milligrams or less per serving. A fast look at the Percent Daily Value will tell you easily if that food is indeed low in sodium (and yet again, there's the famous 5%):

5% OR LESS DAILY VALUE FOR SODIUM

Total Carbohydrate (Including Dietary Fiber and Sugars)

You don't need this part of the label if you're filling up on beans, pasta, vegetables, and fruits (that is, on complex carbohydrates and fiber), because chances are very, very good that you're not eating a whole lot of fatty foods. Cheers! In fact, sugars are not a problem unless you eat all kinds of sugary foods, in which case you probably aren't eating the beans, pasta, vegetables, and fruits just mentioned. What you are doing is paying for your dentist's vacations.[36]

Protein

Y ou'll notice that there's no Percent Daily Value for Protein.[37] It used to be that people didn't eat enough of it, but now just about everybody eats too much.

Vitamins and Minerals

A ccording to the label, Vitamins A and C, plus minerals Calcium and Iron, are the Big Four as far as vitamins and minerals go. If a food contains more than 10 percent of a vitamin or mineral, it is considered a good source.

Now we skip to the very bottom of the label, to:

Calories per Gram

The thing to note here is that a gram of fat has more than twice the calories of a gram of carbohydrate or protein. So, not only is too much fat bad for you, it's FATtening.

Nutrition Facts	
Serving Size 1 cup (228g)	
Servings Per Container 2	

Amount Per Serving	
Calories 260 Calories from Fat 120	

	% Daily Value*
Total Fat 13g	**20%**
Saturated Fat 5g	**25%**
Cholesterol 30mg	**10%**
Sodium 660mg	**28%**
Total Carbohydrate 31g	**10%**
Dietary Fiber 0g	**0%**
Sugars 5g	
Protein 5g	

Vitamin A 4% • Vitamin C 2%
Calcium 15% • Iron 4%

* Percent Daily Values are based on a 2,000 calorie diet. Your daily values may be higher or lower depending on your calorie needs.

		Calories:	2,000	2,500
Total Fat	Less than		65g	80g
Sat Fat	Less than		20g	25g
Cholesterol	Less than		300mg	300mg
Sodium	Less than		2,400mg	2,400mg
Total Carbohydrate			300g	375g
Dietary Fiber			25g	30g

Calories per gram:
Fat 9 • Carbohydrate 4 • Protein 4

How to Use

Food Labels

to Select

Low-Fat Foods

Labels can only do so much.

Looking Back At — And Beyond — The Label

Whether you are following a 10 percent fat diet (exceedingly difficult), a 30 percent fat diet (undoubtedly a happy change from your old habits), or something in between (good for you!), you can use labels as a tool. Maybe it's an imperfect one, but it can remind you of how much fat you take in each day.

If you like to keep careful track of such things, you can use the food labels to *tally grams of fat*. Easier than scoring bowling or bridge.

Or you can *use percentages*. You can tell by the bold typeface that the folks responsible for the food labels (the FDA) are putting a lot of weight behind them. We've seen their usefulness (Percent Daily Value) as a screening tool to choose foods low in Total Fat, Saturated Fat, and Cholesterol, and how the magic 5% quickly identifies these foods.

But life is never perfect, and this is no exception. While labels can tell you whether or not a particular food is low in fat, for example, they can only do so much. Besides, a lot of the food you eat doesn't come in bags or boxes or any other package. You cook, you eat out, you live a life that is largely label free.

Eventually, true knowledge will take over. You won't have to calculate grams of fat, or Percent Daily Value, or anything else, because you will have become so familiar with how things fit together that you will understand the relative place of fat in the diet. You'll know, for example, that there are more and more low-fat and fat-free foods on the market every day. You'll know which cuts of meat are lowest in fat, and that you don't need to eat much of them. You'll know that you'll do better if you avoid cream-based soups, sauces, and gravies, and anything deep fried. An appealing fringe benefit will be that you'll actually feel better when there is less fat in your diet, and you'll very likely come to the point where you find thick, fatty foods unappealing. Tastes do change. When you were a kid, you hated (What? Soup? Potatoes? Vegetables?) and now you're known throughout your zip code for your fabulous minestrone.

Give yourself a chance. It's worth it.

How to Use

Food Labels

to Select

Low-Fat Foods

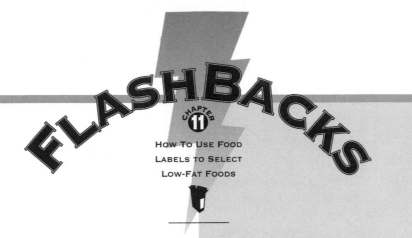

FLASHBACKS

HOW TO USE FOOD
LABELS TO SELECT
LOW-FAT FOODS

☞ Use serving-size information.

☞ **Screen foods for Total Fat, Saturated Fat, and Cholesterol:** NO MORE THAN 5% DAILY VALUE is your guideline.

☞ **Know the Bigger Picture:** According to the label, 65 grams is the Daily Value for fat, although for women that number is probably closer to 50 grams.

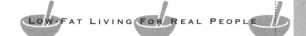
Chapter Twelve
Embarrassingly Simple Recipes

Embarrassingly

Simple

Recipes

Getting Started

This may be a funny thing to say in a book containing recipes, but don't worry too much about following these recipes exactly. Even when they are very, very specific ("4 teaspoons mustard"), that's really only an estimate of how much of a certain ingredient you might like to use. Four teaspoons could be too much, or not enough, or, as Goldilocks may have discovered, just right. To a great extent the amount of garlic, for instance, that you use depends on how much you feel like chopping. So don't be afraid to vary recipes to suit your own taste. On the other hand, if you come upon a recipe for, say, chicken with apricot jam, and you happen to detest apricots, better look for another recipe.

These recipes are all embarrassingly simple. None is simply embarrassing. Some of them hardly deserve to be called recipes at all, but what the heck, we'll call them recipes anyway. They are as close as we could get to what one woman said she was looking for: "Recipes that don't have 'ingredients.'"

Low-fat recipes do, however, follow certain rules, which you'll be applying to recipes wherever you find them. Put these rules together and you wind up with food that is low in total fat as well as saturated fat and cholesterol:

- Servings are held to 3 ounces of Extra Lean meat, fish, or poultry.
- If dairy products are used, they are low fat or fat free.
- If fat is added, it is monounsaturated (olive or canola oil).
- Added fat is held to one teaspoon per serving. This rule may be broken for real salad dressing (see recipe for Our Favorite Oil and Vinegar Dressing, page 174) or for an occasional real treat (see recipe for Vanilla Soufflé to Remember, page 188), but always with an eye on The Bigger Picture.

Nutrient analysis is a standard part of recipes nowadays, and we have included the calories, fat, carbohydrate, protein, and sodium per serving in each recipe given here. Because these are heart-healthy recipes, the nutrient levels stay within the guidelines suggested by the label law.[38] And we have provided "sodium alerts"[39] for those on sodium-restricted diets.

You'll notice that these recipes make use of special flavor enhancers – broth, wine, yogurt, and tomatoes. We don't want low fat to be synonymous with low flavor.

You'll notice that several soups are included. You might not consider making your own soup to be embarrassingly simple, but these soups are very hearty. All you have to add is salad, bread, and fruit to turn them into lunch or supper, and that makes them very convenient. (Imagine – making your own soup and finding that you've actually saved time!) We prefer to think of them as "floating casseroles." Like ordinary casseroles, they can be made ahead and reheated when needed.

And you'll notice that there are no meat recipes. You've been cooking embarrassingly simple meat recipes for years (also known as throwing hamburgers on the grill), and you don't need to hear more about that here. Besides, as we have noted before, people have chosen chicken as a kind of "transition food" in an effort to eat low fat. We therefore offer chicken recipes, fish recipes, plus quite a number that contain neither chicken nor fish.

Low fat doesn't have to mean low flavor.

No-Fat Flavor Enhancers

CHICKEN BROTH: Chicken broth is an embarrassingly simple, nonfat (*assuming you take the fat off*) flavor-enhancer. The downside is that the convenient canned versions tend to be high in salt, but the upside is that there are lower salt versions available as well.

> **BEST HOT TIP OF THE DECADE AND WELL WORTH REPEATING:**
>
> Store canned chicken broth in the refrigerator. All the fat will congeal on top, just begging to be removed in an unattractive lump and thrown away.

VEGETABLE BROTH: Swanson makes a canned, clear vegetable broth that is very, very low in fat (but high in salt, so a little goes a long way) and is full of flavor. And if the food you cook has a lot of flavor, you won't miss the fat you've eliminated.

WINE provides excellent, no-fat flavor, with most (but not all) of the alcohol evaporating during cooking. And how's this for a "seal of approval"? Wine is used in more than a few of the recipes in *The American Heart Association Low-Fat, Low-Cholesterol Cookbook.*

YOGURT: Ah, cream, the basis for many fine, rich foods – and heart disease. For a creamy texture without a medical alert, use nonfat yogurt. It is a chameleon that, seasoned with herbs and spices, or with mustard added, becomes a flavorful marinade, dip, or dressing. (By the way, check labels and pick a mustard with no fat in it. In particular, mustards with horseradish, or that call themselves "creamy," tend to contain fat.)

> ### TO THICKEN YOGURT:
> Put a coffee filter in a strainer, then put the strainer over a bowl. Fill strainer with plain, nonfat yogurt. Cover and put the whole thing in the refrigerator. The longer you leave it there, the thicker the yogurt will get. Twenty minutes will see some results, but if you leave it for several hours or overnight, you'll be left with yogurt that is thick and cream cheese-like. Mixed with a little mustard, it is wonderful to use on sandwiches instead of mayonnaise.

TOMATOES: All sorts of tomato products enhance flavors wonderfully and you'll find that a number of the following recipes make use of tomatoes. Those that call for tomato sauce or crushed tomatoes manage to deliver a lot of sodium along with flavor, so if you are cutting back on sodium, look for low-sodium versions in the supermarket. (Low-sodium alternative brands are suggested along with the recipes.) Fresh and sun-dried tomatoes are not high in sodium.

Making Food Juicy Without Fat

MARINATING: By soaking food in something before you cook it, you make it juicier, tastier, and more tender. Plain, nonfat yogurt can be flavored with herbs and spices or mustard, thus miraculously becoming a nonfat marinade. So does fat-free salad dressing, available in every supermarket. (Choose low-sodium versions if you are restricting sodium.) Wine, which is fat free, makes a fine marinade, too.

All marinating has in common the fact that the process goes on without you. Just get things going in the morning, even the night before, and when it comes time to do the cooking, great things will have happened in your absence.

USING FOIL: You can make foods juicy by adding liquid – broth, wine, or crushed tomatoes in juice, for example – and sealing with foil. Foil allows food to steam in the flavorful juices. It also makes cleanup embarrassingly simple.

◆   ◆   ◆   ◆

Occasionally you may want to use just a bit of fat in your cooking, in which case you can *sauté*. High heat makes a *small amount of fat* in the pan go a long way. Sauté means "jump" in French, and you don't need much fat to make that happen. In fact, you can buy cooking oil in a spray can, then spray a very, very light coating in a non-stick skillet (just a puff, really), and get away with a whole lot less fat. This fast cooking gives foods – sliced mushrooms, say – an entirely different (and delicious) flavor.

Here we go.

Chicken

(with one turkey recipe for good measure)

Now come the EMBARRASSINGLY SIMPLE chicken recipes. Various things happen to the chicken. Each recipe serves four and therefore requires four small halves of boneless, skinless chicken breasts. These serving sizes are probably smaller than you are used to. When you are at the supermarket, standing in front of the poultry case, look for a package that contains 4 such breasts, for a total weight of 1 pound. When cooked, the breasts will weigh about 3 ounces each.

"Roadrunner"
4 Servings

Olive oil is the only added fat in this recipe. Crushed tomatoes and lemon juice, of course, contain no fat, and provide the flavorful liquid in which the chicken "steams."

4 small (4-ounce) halves chicken breast, boneless and skinless

Mrs. Dash or other dried herb seasoning

1 small onion, chopped

1 clove garlic, minced fine (or use the garlic that comes in a cute little jar, all ready to use)

2 teaspoons olive oil

1 teaspoon lemon juice

1 14-ounce can crushed tomatoes

Preheat oven to 350°F.

Rinse chicken under cold running water. Pat dry with paper towel and lay in baking dish in single layer. Season to taste with the dried herb seasoning.

Using a small, nonstick skillet, sauté onion and garlic in olive oil until translucent. Sprinkle on top of chicken. Add lemon juice to crushed tomatoes and pour over all. Cover with foil and bake for 45 minutes.

Per Serving:
Calories: 193   **Fat:** 5g **Carbohydrate:** 8g
Protein: 27g   **Sodium:** 350mg

SODIUM ALERT!
If you are on a sodium-restricted diet, then use, for example, Eden "no salt added" crushed tomatoes.

Embarrassingly

Simple

Recipes

Chicken with Sun-dried Tomato Paste
4 Servings

Cooking with wine is one of the fat-free cooking methods. And foil keeps the chicken juicy.

4 small (4-ounce) halves chicken breast, boneless and skinless
4 teaspoons sun-dried tomato paste (see recipe, page 176)
1/4 cup white wine
Heavy aluminum foil large enough to make envelope around chicken

Preheat oven to 350°F.

Rinse chicken breasts in cold water; pat dry with paper towel. Lay in single layer on foil. Spread sun-dried tomato paste on each piece, pour wine around chicken, seal foil, place in a baking dish, and bake for 45 minutes.

Per Serving:
Calories: 193   **Fat:** 5g **Carbohydrate:** 8g **Protein:** 27g **Sodium:** 63mg

All-Purpose Chicken

4 Servings

This is a pleasantly moist, plain chicken that may be used "as is," and is also wonderful for all sorts of other things: chicken salad, sandwiches, and as a topping for a green salad.

You'll see that this recipe bears a startling resemblance to Chicken with Sun-dried Tomato Paste, but that's the way it is with these things. When you are cooking embarrassingly simple food, you find that minor recipe changes result in major taste differences.

> **4 small (4-ounce) halves chicken breast, boneless and skinless**
>
> **Mrs. Dash or other dried herb mixture (*OR* chili powder *OR* curry powder if you prefer)**
>
> **Heavy aluminum foil large enough to make envelope around chicken**

Preheat oven to 350°F.

Rinse chicken breasts in cold water; pat dry with paper towel. Lay in single layer on foil. Sprinkle with the dried herb mixture OR the chili powder OR the curry powder, seal foil, place in a baking dish and bake for 45 minutes.

Per Serving:
Calories: 135   **Fat:** 3g   **Carbohydrate:** 0g   **Protein:** 27g   **Sodium:** 63mg

Embarrassingly

Simple

Recipes

Unlikely Chicken
4 Servings

As long as you use mustard made without oil, this recipe contains no added fat. It does, however, contain some ingredients that look rather – ahem – strange. Just goes to show that you can't always judge a recipe by reading it!

> **4 small (4-ounce) halves chicken breast, boneless and skinless**
> **1/3 cup nonfat plain yogurt**
> **1/3 cup apricot or raspberry all-fruit preserves**
> **1 tablespoon Dijon mustard**

Preheat oven to 350°F.

Rinse chicken breasts in cold water; pat dry with paper towel. Place in a small, shallow baking dish in a single layer. Combine yogurt, preserves, and mustard (we know, we know, but trust us), spread over the chicken breasts, and bake uncovered for 45 minutes.

Per Serving:
Calories: 219 **Fat:** 3g **Carbohydrate:** 21g **Protein:** 27g **Sodium:** 83mg

Chicken Marinated in Yogurt
4 Servings

Because you are using nonfat yogurt, there's no added fat in this recipe. Also you'll see that yogurt makes a great marinade and gives the cooked chicken a nice brown crust.

> **4 small (4-ounce) halves chicken breast, boneless and skinless**
> **1/2 cup nonfat plain yogurt**
> **1 clove garlic, chopped fine (or use the garlic that comes in a cute little jar, all ready to use)**
> **1 teaspoon dried mint**
> **Freshly ground pepper to taste**

Rinse chicken breasts in cold water; pat dry with paper towel. Combine yogurt, garlic, and mint in a bowl. Add chicken, tossing to coat well with yogurt. Add pepper and stir well. Refrigerate several hours or overnight, allowing to marinate. When dinnertime rolls around, as it has a way of doing, broil 7 minutes on each side.

Per Serving:
Calories: 151 **Fat:** 3g **Carbohydrate:** 2g **Protein:** 29g **Sodium:** 88mg

Embarrassingly

Simple

Recipes

Grilled Turkey Breast
4 Servings

The boneless, skinless turkey breast has come to the supermarket. It makes a nice change from the usual roasted affair, the recipe for which you can find in more than a few cookbooks. This recipe looks longer than the others but it's still very easy. Yogurt is used as a marinade, which moistens and flavors the turkey while you're off doing something else.

In order to make 4 servings, you need a 1-pound package of boneless turkey breast, but you will probably only find one that weighs a bit more, maybe "1.33 pounds" or so. This will give you leftovers to add to Updated Pasta Salad (see recipe, page 168).

1 1-pound package turkey breast (weight approximate), boneless and skinless

1 tablespoon lemon juice

MARINADE:

1 cup plain, nonfat yogurt

1 teaspoon celery seed

2 garlic cloves, crushed (or use the garlic that comes in a cute little jar, all ready to use)

1/2 teaspoon freshly ground pepper

Other herbs and spices of your choice (optional)

When you get home and take the turkey breast out of the package, it won't look wildly appetizing, but don't despair. Rinse it in cold water, then pat dry with paper towel. Cut two little slashes in turkey and put it in a flat baking dish. Put a bit of the lemon juice in each slash. Some will spill over, but don't worry about that.

Combine marinade ingredients and coat the turkey. Cover and refrigerate, allowing to marinate for several hours or overnight, turning once. (No need to set your alarm to wake you in the middle of the night. Flip it when you get up for breakfast.) Then cook on a grill (with a hood), for 30 minutes, turning once. Keep hood closed while turkey is cooking. If your grill has a heat adjustment, use "medium." If not, set the rack a bit away from the coals.

If you don't have access to a grill, you can broil the turkey breast instead, probably about 20 minutes on each side, but the time will depend on thickness. The breast is done when you poke a fork into it and the juices run clear, not pink.

When the turkey is completely cooked, allow to cool for a few minutes to make slicing easier. Also good served at room temperature.

Per Serving:
Calories: 183 **Fat:** 3g **Carbohydrate:** 5g **Protein:** 34g **Sodium:** 104mg

Embarrassingly

Simple

Recipes

Fish

Fish is wonderful for a low-fat diet and offers welcome variety. Note that timing is important when cooking fish, and that cooking any fish too long results in something that is dry, firm, tasteless, and generally just plain unappealing.

Carefree Flounder

4 Servings

This recipe uses lemon juice and wine, neither of which contains fat. Ditto mustard (such as Grey Poupon Dijon). The most time-consuming part of the recipe is unwrapping the fish.

1 pound fresh flounder fillets
4 teaspoons Dijon mustard
2 tablespoons lemon juice
1/3 cup white wine

Preheat oven to 350°F.

Lay the flounder in a single layer in a baking dish. Spread with mustard. Pour lemon juice and wine over all, and bake for 20 minutes. (If this strikes you as being just a little too simple, cut up a carrot, a medium tomato, and half a small onion. Put on top of fish before you put it in the oven.)

Per Serving:
Calories: 124 **Fat:** 1g **Carbohydrate:** 1g **Protein:** 17g **Sodium:** 126mg

Embarrassingly

Simple

Recipes

Salmon Cooked in Foil
4 Servings

Cooking in foil holds in juices and has the added advantage of leaving you with a pan that needs little or no scrubbing.

1 pound fresh salmon fillet (ask to have any large bones removed)

1 scallion, chopped

4 pieces sun-dried tomatoes that come marinated in olive oil; drained well and blotted with paper towels, then snipped in strips

1 tablespoon fresh tarragon (or other herb of your choice), snipped in small pieces

1/4 cup dry white wine

Freshly ground pepper to taste

Heavy aluminum foil, large enough to make an envelope around fish

Preheat oven to 450°F.

Lay salmon on foil. Sprinkle with scallion, sun-dried tomatoes, and tarragon (or other herb). Grind fresh pepper over all. Carefully pour wine over fish, seal aluminum pouch, lay in ovenproof dish and bake for 25 minutes.

Per Serving:
Calories: 198 **Fat:** 7g **Carbohydrate:** 3g **Protein:** 22g **Sodium:** 85mg

VARIATION: Lay the salmon on foil, sprinkle with 1 tablespoon fines herbes, dried, and freshly ground pepper. Seal foil and cook as above. (This is so good cold that you might want to just prepare it ahead and refrigerate, foil and all, for later use. Delicious served with Yogurt-Mustard Sauce, see recipe, page 177).

Per Serving:
Calories: 151 **Fat:** 7g **Carbohydrate:** 0g **Protein:** 22g **Sodium:** 48mg

Baked Mackerel

4 Servings

Marinating for even a short time makes the fish especially moist and flavorful.

1 pound fresh mackerel fillets
2 tablespoons lemon juice
1/2 teaspoon dried rosemary
1/2 teaspoon dried thyme
Freshly ground pepper to taste

Place fish in single layer, skin side down, in a shallow baking dish. Drizzle lemon juice over fish; sprinkle with herbs and fresh pepper. Cover dish with foil and refrigerate for an hour or more. About 30 minutes before you plan to start cooking, set the dish on the counter.

Preheat oven to 450°F.

Bake for 20 minutes.

Per Serving:
Calories: 125   **Fat:** 5g   **Carbohydrate:** 0g   **Protein:** 20g   **Sodium:** 56mg

Embarrassingly

Simple

Recipes

Shrimp with Tomatoes
4 Servings

You'll want to use fresh, not frozen, shrimp for this.   Shrimp is very low in fat and, in moderate amounts, good for a heart-healthy diet. Serving the shrimp and tomatoes over rice helps to keep the amount moderate. While you're at it, why not try brown rice, which has the well-earned reputation of being particularly good for you? If you think of brown rice as being sticky and chewy, try Uncle Ben's Original Brown rice. It is neither of the above, and it tastes very good.

> **1/4 cup lemon juice**
> **2 teaspoons olive oil**
> **2 cloves garlic, crushed (or use the garlic that comes in a cute little jar, all ready to use)**
> **1 pound medium fresh shrimp, peeled (about 32 shrimp)**
> **1 28-ounce can crushed tomatoes**
> **Freshly ground pepper to taste**

Combine lemon juice, olive oil, and garlic in a small bowl. Toss with shrimp. Cover with plastic wrap. Allow to marinate several hours in the refrigerator. (If you decide late in the day to make this, set bowl on counter for 1/2 hour before cooking.)

Remove shrimp from marinade and add liquid to tomatoes. Heat tomato mixture in a medium saucepan. While it is heating, cook shrimp by stir-frying them in a well-heated nonstick skillet for about 3 minutes or so. Allow to brown slightly. Add to tomatoes and season with pepper. Serve over rice.

Per Serving (without rice):
Calories: 147   **Fat:** 3g **Carbohydrate:** 10g
Protein: 20g   **Sodium:** 570mg

SODIUM ALERT!

If you are on a sodium-restricted diet, then substitute, for example, Eden "no salt added" crushed tomatoes.

Crunchy Tuna Salad

(Or use canned red salmon to make Salmon Salad)

2 Servings

1 6½-ounce can solid white tuna in water

2 tablespoons canned water chestnuts, chopped

1 small carrot, chopped, about 1/8 cup

2 teaspoons red onion, chopped

1 tablespoon chopped celery

1/4 cup nonfat plain yogurt

1 teaspoon Dijon mustard

Drain tuna, empty into a bowl, and mash with fork. Add water chestnuts, carrot, red onion and celery. Mix together. Combine yogurt and mustard, then add to tuna salad.

Per Serving:

Calories: 134   **Fat:** 2g **Carbohydrate:** 5g
Protein: 24g **Sodium:** 389mg

> **SODIUM ALERT!**
>
> If you are on a sodium-restricted diet, use a tuna such as Bumble Bee Diet Low Salt Chunk White Tuna packed in water, or Chicken of the Sea Diet Chunk Light Tuna packed in water.

> **SODIUM ALERT!**
>
> If you are on a sodium-restricted diet, use a salmon such as Season Blueback or Pink Salmon, "no salt added," or Featherweight Pink Salmon, "no salt added."

If made with salmon:

Per Serving:

Calories: 196   **Fat:** 7g   **Carbohydrate:** 9g
Protein: 24g   **Sodium:** 552mg

Embarrassingly

Simple

Recipes

Vegetables

We've come a long way since vegetables were an afterthought, and they can be a remarkable addition to a meal. We have a number of suggestions as to how to cook vegetables; some recipes use no fat at all. Remember, as you develop your own recipes, think "no more than 1 teaspoon (5 grams) of added fat per serving."

Vegetable Combo
6 Servings

It's possible to brown foods without fat, and this recipe shows you how. Try other vegetables – bell peppers, for instance – the next time you make this.

1/4 cup Swanson's Clear Vegetable Broth or other fat-free broth
1 medium white onion (sweet), sliced
1 medium zucchini, cubed
1 medium yellow (summer) squash, cubed
6 fairly large fresh mushrooms, sliced
1 teaspoon fines herbes, dried
4 fresh medium plum tomatoes, cut up
Freshly ground pepper to taste

Put broth and onion in a large, nonstick skillet and simmer until onion is transparent. Add squash and mushrooms. Sprinkle with fines herbes. Let cook until liquid evaporates and vegetables start to brown a bit, about 10 to 15 minutes. Keep heat high and DON'T LEAVE THE PREMISES! Stir from time to time. Add tomatoes and stir as they cook into the vegetable mixture. Season with fresh pepper.

Per Serving:
Calories: 28 **Fat:** 0g **Carbohydrate:** 5g **Protein:** 2g **Sodium:** 77mg

Embarrassingly

Simple

Recipes

Fresh Spinach and Portobello Mushrooms
4 Servings

If you're lucky, you'll be able to find that the spinach in a cellophane bag has been pre-washed. If so, add 1/4 cup of water to the skillet when you add the spinach. Otherwise, when you wash it, enough water will cling to the leaves to make the extra water unnecessary.

1 teaspoon olive oil

2 large cloves garlic, chopped (or use the garlic that comes in a cute little jar, all ready to use)

1 medium onion, chopped

6 ounces fresh Portobello mushrooms, sliced

1 10-ounce package fresh spinach in cellophane, washed

Freshly ground pepper to taste

Heat olive oil in a large, nonstick skillet. Add garlic and onion; cook until translucent. Add mushroom slices and cook over medium heat until very soft, about 10 minutes. Add spinach (as well as extra water, if necessary). Cover with lid or foil. Allow to steam for another 10 minutes or so, until spinach is wilted but still bright green. Season with pepper and stir well.

Per Serving:
Calories: 50 **Fat:** 2g **Carbohydrate:** 5g **Protein:** 3g **Sodium:** 64mg

Mushrooms in Foil
4 Servings

Incredibly easy, no cleanup, and perfect as a side dish or as a "sauce" for fish or chicken. There's no need to add any liquid, because, as you'll see, the mushrooms have lots of juice.

> **1 pound fresh mushrooms (mix varieties if desired)**
> **Freshly ground pepper to taste**
> **Dried herb of your choice, such as oregano (optional)**
> **Foil**

Preheat oven to 400°F.

Slice mushrooms and lay on foil. Sprinkle with pepper (and herbs, if you've decided to use them). Seal foil and bake for 15 to 20 minutes.

Per Serving:
Calories: 36 **Fat:** 0g **Carbohydrate:** 5g **Protein:** 4g **Sodium:** 20mg

Embarrassingly

Simple

Recipes

Savoy Cabbage with Carrots
4 Servings

Even if you aren't a big cabbage fan, give savoy cabbage a try. Its flavor is much more delicate than that of the original.

> **1 small head savoy cabbage**
>
> **1 13 3/4-ounce can chicken broth (College Inn Lower Salt. Chill can for easy removal of fat.)**
>
> **1/2 package small, peeled carrots (available in supermarket produce section)**
>
> **1 teaspoon caraway seeds (optional)**

Cut cabbage in quarters; remove core and discard. Rinse cabbage and slice thin. Put cabbage in a medium saucepan with the broth and carrots. Bring to a boil and reduce heat. Simmer, covered, until vegetables are tender, about 30 minutes. Sprinkle with caraway seeds if you feel like it.

Per Serving:
Calories: 77 **Fat:** 1g **Carbohydrate:** 13g
Protein: 4g   **Sodium:** 275mg

> **SODIUM ALERT!**
>
> If you are on a sodium-restricted diet, then substitute, for example, Health Valley "no salt added" chicken broth.

"Mexican" Eggplant
4 Servings

Again, a casserole, convenient in that it can be fixed ahead.

1 15-ounce can tomato sauce

1 small to medium eggplant, unpeeled and sliced on the diagonal, giving you bigger, easier-to-layer slices

1/2 pound fresh mushrooms, sliced

1 medium white sweet onion, sliced

1 16-ounce can of pink (or other) beans, rinsed, drained, and puréed with 1/2 can of water

1/2 teaspoon dried cumin, puréed with beans (optional)

2 tablespoons chopped fresh chives (optional)

Preheat oven to 350°F.

Spread a bit of the tomato sauce in the bottom of a shallow baking dish (13 1/2" x 8 3/4" x 1 3/4"), and then start layering. First, the slices of eggplant. Then scatter some mushrooms and onion slices around. Add more of the tomato sauce. Make another layer of eggplant, mushroom, and onion slices. Before adding more tomato sauce, spread the puréed beans (that have been combined with cumin, if desired) and then top with the sauce. Bake for one hour, or until bubbly. Sprinkle fresh chives on top if you are using them.

Per Serving:
Calories: 167   **Fat:** 1g   **Carbohydrate:** 30g
Protein: 9g   **Sodium:** 710mg

> **SODIUM ALERT!**
>
> If you are on a sodium-restricted diet, then use, for example, Hunt's "no salt added" tomato sauce and Eden "very low sodium" canned beans.

Eggplant and Tomato

(puréed and delicious)

4 Servings

1 large eggplant

1 small onion, chopped fine

1 clove garlic, chopped fine (or use the garlic that comes in a cute little jar, all ready to use)

1/4 cup chopped fresh parsley

1 large tomato, peeled and chopped (Dip tomato briefly in boiling water; it will peel easily.)

1 tablespoon lemon juice

Freshly ground pepper to taste

Preheat oven to 450°F.

Pierce eggplant with a fork and bake until very soft, about 1/2 hour. While eggplant is cooking, put onion, garlic, parsley, and tomato in a small, nonstick skillet lightly sprayed with oil. Cook slowly until vegetables are soft.

When eggplant is fully cooked, allow to cool before handling, unless you are blessed with asbestos hands. Then cut it in half lengthwise and scrape pulp out of shell into bowl of food processor. Add vegetables and purée the whole thing. Stir in lemon juice and pepper. Serve hot or cold, either as a side dish or an hors d'oeuvre, spread on crackers.

Per Serving:
Calories: 48 **Fat:** 0g **Carbohydrate:** 10g   **Protein:** 2g **Sodium:** 6mg

Rice, Pasta, Potatoes, Barley, and Beans

Embarrassingly

Simple

Recipes

Embarrassingly

Simple

Recipes

Rice, Pasta, and Spinach — Together at Last
4 Servings

In this recipe you want to brown the rice and spaghetti before they start to cook. As you can see, when you use a nonstick skillet you need very little oil. (In fact, you can often get away with none at all.)

If you prefer, you can make this without the spinach. We know a nine-year-old who won't eat much of anything but loves the spinach-free version.

1 teaspoon olive oil

1 medium onion, chopped

3/4 cup uncooked rice

1/4 cup uncooked thin spaghetti, broken in 1-inch pieces

1 13 3/4-ounce can defatted chicken broth (College Inn Lower Salt. Chill can for easy removal of fat.)

3/4 cup water

1 package frozen spinach, thawed and drained (to thaw, run under cold water)

Using a large, nonstick skillet, heat the oil and cook onion until transparent. Add rice and pasta. Stir until lightly browned. Add broth and water and bring to a boil. Reduce heat, cover with lid or foil, and cook for 15 minutes. Stir in spinach with fork, cover again, and cook until liquid is absorbed, about 15 minutes more.

Per Serving:
Calories: 148 **Fat:** 2g **Carbohydrate:** 26g
Protein: 7g   **Sodium:** 395mg

> **SODIUM ALERT!**
>
> If you are on a sodium-restricted diet, then substitute, for example, Health Valley "no salt added" chicken broth.

Barley and Tomatoes with Apples

(if you can imagine)

4 Servings

If you've never used barley before, you'll find it in the supermarket with the rice and dried beans. It comes in a box or a plastic bag, your choice.

1 28-ounce can tomatoes, drained and chopped

1 13 3/4-ounce can defatted chicken broth (College Inn Lower Salt. Chill can for easy removal of fat.)

1 1/4 cups water

1 cup barley

1 medium onion, chopped

3 medium Granny Smith apples, peeled, cored, and sliced thin, about 2 cups

Put tomatoes, broth, and water in a large saucepan. Bring to a boil. Add barley and chopped onion, reduce heat, cover, and cook for 30 minutes. Add apples. Cook another 15 minutes, until liquid is absorbed.

Per Serving:

Calories: 205   **Fat:** 1g   **Carbohydrate:** 46g
Protein: 3g   **Sodium:** 660mg

> **SODIUM ALERT!**
>
> If you are on a sodium-restricted diet, use, for example, Eden "no salt added" canned tomatoes, and substitute, for example, Health Valley "no salt added" chicken broth.

Embarrassingly

Simple

Recipes

Not Too Boring Potato-Onion Casserole
4 Servings

Not only does this recipe have no added fat, but, because it's a casserole, it can be prepared ahead and cooked at dinner time.

> **4 medium Idaho potatoes**
> **2 medium onions**
> **1 teaspoon dried basil**
> **1 teaspoon dried, crushed bay leaf**
> **1 13 3/4-ounce can defatted chicken broth (College Inn Lower Salt. Chill can for easy removal of fat.)**
> **Mrs. Dash or other dried herb seasoning**

Preheat oven to 400°F.

Peel potatoes and slice thin. Put in cold water. Cut onions in thin slices. Using a shallow baking dish that can be placed on the stovetop, layer potatoes, onions, basil, and bay leaf. Continue to layer until used up.

Pour chicken broth over the top. Sprinkle with herb seasoning. Bring to a boil on the stove, cover with foil, reduce heat, and simmer for 5 minutes. Put in oven and bake, uncovered, for 25 minutes.

Per Serving:
Calories: 137 **Fat:** 1g **Carbohydrate:** 28g
Protein: 4g **Sodium:** 275mg

> ### SODIUM ALERT!
> If you are on a sodium-restricted diet, then substitute, for example, Health Valley "no salt added" chicken broth.

Sweet Potato "Chips"
4 Servings

This is a taste treat that is easy to prepare because you don't have to peel the potatoes.

2 large unpeeled, sweet potatoes, sliced thin (the thinner the slice, the crisper the chip)
Cayenne pepper
   OR **paprika**
   OR **chili powder**

Preheat oven to 450°F.

Place sweet potato slices in single layer on nonstick cookie sheet (recipe will make two batches). For a touch of spice, sprinkle lightly with ONE of the suggested options. Bake 15 minutes, flipping once during baking. Remove from oven when chips are nicely browned. (The exact cooking time will depend on the thickness of the chips; keep an eye on them so they don't burn.) May be served hot or cold.

Per Serving:
Calories: 125 **Fat:** 1g **Carbohydrate:** 27g **Protein:** 2g **Sodium:** 11mg

Embarrassingly

Simple

Recipes

Embarrassingly Simple Rice

4 Servings

> **1 13 3/4-ounce can defatted chicken broth (College Inn Lower Salt. Chill can for easy removal of fat.)**
> **3/4 cup water**
> **1/2 teaspoon dried thyme**
> **1 medium onion, cut up**
> **1 cup white rice**

Put the broth and water in a medium saucepan and bring to a boil. Stir in thyme, onion, and rice, cover, and lower the heat. Cook over moderate heat until liquid is absorbed, about 25 minutes.

SODIUM ALERT!

If you are on a sodium-restricted diet, then substitute, for example, Health Valley "no salt added" chicken broth.

Per Serving:

Calories: 104   **Fat:** 0g **Carbohydrate:** 23g
Protein: 3g   **Sodium:** 275mg

Interesting variation: In food processor, put 6 fresh mushrooms that have been washed and dried. Process them so that they are chopped very, very fine. Put them in a large, nonstick skillet. Add two table-spoons of water and cook over low heat, letting the juices escape. When the chopped mushrooms are dry, stir while they brown slightly. Add them to the broth and water (with the thyme and onions if you like), stir, then add the rice and cook as directed above. To be a little fancier, buy one of the wild rice/white rice blends that are on the market. Adjust amount of liquid according to the directions on the package. (This is a remarkable dish for company.)

Per Serving:

Calories: 104 **Fat:** 0g **Carbohydrate:** 24g **Protein:** 3g **Sodium:** 276mg

(Same sodium alert!)

Jack Sprat's Rice with Black Beans

4 Servings

1 13 3/4-ounce can defatted chicken broth (College Inn Lower Salt. Chill can for easy removal of fat.)

1/4 cup water

1/2 cup white wine

1 small onion, chopped

1 medium carrot, scraped and chopped

3/4 cup uncooked rice

1/2 16-ounce can black beans, rinsed well

Put broth, water, wine, onion, and carrot in a medium saucepan and bring to a boil. Add rice and beans, cover, and reduce heat. Cook until liquid is absorbed, about 30 minutes. (This can also be done in the oven, which is handy if your oven is the kind that will turn itself on before you get home. Just put everything in a 2-quart baking dish and set the timer so the rice and beans will bake for one hour at 350°F.)

SODIUM ALERT!

If you are on a sodium-restricted diet, then substitute, for example, Health Valley "no salt added" chicken broth and use, for example, Eden "very low sodium" canned beans.

Per Serving:
Calories: 177 **Fat:** 1g **Carbohydrate:** 37g
Protein: 5g **Sodium:** 390mg

Embarrassingly

Simple

Recipes

Chickpeas (Garbanzo Beans), Fast and Furious
4 Servings

Even if the idea of eating beans has never appealed to you, you might try this recipe. In just a couple of minutes you'll have a delicious side dish.

> **2 teaspoons olive oil**
> **1 medium onion, cut up**
> **2 cloves garlic, chopped fine (or use the garlic that comes in a cute little jar, all ready to use)**
> **1 16-ounce can chickpeas, drained and rinsed well**
> **Freshly ground pepper to taste**

Heat the olive oil in a medium, nonstick skillet over moderate heat. Add the onion and garlic and sauté until translucent. Add chickpeas, toss quickly to heat through, and finish off with a dose of freshly ground pepper.

Per Serving:
Calories: 136   **Fat:** 4g   **Carbohydrate:** 19g
Protein: 6g   **Sodium:** 180mg

> ### SODIUM ALERT!
>
> If you are on a sodium-restricted diet, then use, for example, Eden "very low sodium" canned beans.

Rice and Green Pea Salad

6 Servings

This is a no-fat-added salad with a twist.

> **3/4 cup uncooked rice**
> **2 cups water**
> **1/4 cup lemon juice**
> **1 teaspoon mustard**
> **1 10-ounce box frozen peas, thawed but not cooked**

Cook rice in water according to directions. Cool. Mix lemon juice and mustard together and mix into rice. Add peas.

Per Serving:
Calories: 84   **Fat:** 0g   **Carbohydrate:** 18g   **Protein:** 3g   **Sodium:** 85mg

Embarrassingly

Simple

Recipes

Embarrassingly

Simple

Recipes

Peas of Summer
3 Servings

Best made whenever you can get fresh mint.

1 10-ounce box frozen peas
1/4 cup fresh mint leaves, finely chopped

Cook peas according to directions on package. Drain. Stir in chopped mint and serve promptly.

Per Serving:
Calories: 64 **Fat:** 0g **Carbohydrate:** 12g **Protein:** 4g **Sodium:** 70mg

Marinated Beans and Vegetables

4 Servings

Embarrassingly

Simple

Recipes

1 10-ounce box frozen mixed vegetables

1 16-ounce can chickpeas or other beans, rinsed and drained

2 tablespoons red onion, chopped fine

1/4 cup Pritikin Fat-Free Dijon Balsamic or Fat-Free Honey French bottled dressing

Empty vegetables into a strainer and rinse with cold water. Put in a bowl with beans and onion. Pour dressing over all and mix well. Cover and allow to marinate for an hour or more on the counter, or overnight in the refrigerator.

Per Serving:

Calories: 193 **Fat:** 1g **Carbohydrate:** 37g
Protein: 9g **Sodium:** 260mg

SODIUM ALERT!

If you are on a sodium-restricted diet, then use, for example, Eden "very low sodium" canned beans.

Embarrassingly

Simple

Recipes

Updated Pasta Salad
4 Servings

Happily, fat is not an issue with pasta. And, because all pastas are made from pretty much the same ingredients and differ only in their shape, you can easily vary the look of your pasta dishes.

This is a good summer dish, best served at room temperature, and can be made ahead. Water chestnuts provide a nice crunch, and they don't contain fat. The dressing called for is Wish-Bone Lite Classic Dijon Vinaigrette, a bottled dressing with half the fat of regular. Because it is not fat free, it has not sacrificed taste.

A few slices of leftover Grilled Turkey Breast (see recipe, page 142) are a nice addition to this salad.

> **1/2 of a 1-pound box interestingly shaped pasta, such as rotini or cavatelli, cooked just until done and rinsed to remove starch**
>
> **8 cherry tomatoes, halved**
>
> **1/2 8-ounce can sliced water chestnuts, drained**
>
> **4 leaves fresh basil, chopped**
>
> **2 tablespoons red onion, chopped**
>
> **2 leaves raw spinach, washed, stems removed, and cut up with scissors**
>
> **4 large black olives, sliced thin**
>
> **1/2 cup Wish-Bone Lite Classic Dijon Vinaigrette**

Place pasta, cherry tomatoes, water chestnuts, basil, red onion, spinach and olives in a large bowl. Toss with dressing.

If you are making this ahead, refrigerate. Allow to return to room temperature before serving.

Per Serving:
Calories: 279   **Fat:** 7g **Carbohydrate:** 47g
Protein: 7g   **Sodium:** 393mg

SODIUM ALERT!
If you are on a sodium-restricted diet, use a low-sodium, fat-free dressing, and skip the olives.

Embarrassingly

Simple

Recipes

"Floating Casseroles," Et Cetera

We remind you that floating casseroles are hearty soups that, with the addition of salad, bread, and fruit, serve nicely as lunch or supper. Like casseroles, they can be made ahead and reheated at meal time.

Embarrassingly

Simple

Recipes

Vegetable Soup with Puréed Beans
Floating Casserole I
4 Servings

This soup is just the thing to get non-bean-eaters to eat beans. The beans are puréed and blended into the soup, and no one knows they are there. (Here we have suggested using low-sodium canned beans, so that the per-serving sodium level of the soup will not be unacceptably high.)

1 14-ounce package soup vegetables (celery, parsnip, turnip, carrot, parsley, dill, et cetera, conveniently packaged and waiting for you in the produce section of your supermarket)

2 13 3/4-ounce cans defatted chicken broth (College Inn Lower Salt. Chill can for easy removal of fat.)

1/2 cup water

1 16-ounce can very low sodium navy beans, such as Eden, drained and rinsed

Rinse, peel (as necessary), and chop all vegetables. Place in a large saucepan. Add broth. Bring to a boil, then simmer, covered, until tender, about 30 minutes. Meanwhile, add the water to the beans and purée in a food processor. At the end of the 30 minutes, add to the soup for thickening and great taste. Simmer 15 minutes longer.

Per Serving:
Calories: 184 **Fat:** 0g **Carbohydrate:** 38g
Protein: 8g   **Sodium:** 593mg

SODIUM ALERT!

If you are on a sodium-restricted diet, then substitute, for example, Health Valley "no salt added" chicken broth.

Bean and Pasta Soup
Floating Casserole II
8 servings

This recipe calls for frozen spinach, which means you don't have to take the time to pick off the tough stems and then get the sand out of the leaves, but if you'd rather use fresh, that's great.

3 13 3/4-ounce cans defatted chicken broth (College Inn Lower Salt. Chill cans for easy removal of fat. Save cans for measuring water.)

3 cans water

1/2 16-ounce box "ditalini" pasta (tiny pasta tubes)

1 16-ounce can white kidney beans, drained and rinsed well

1 box frozen leaf spinach, thawed and drained (to thaw, put in colander and run under cold water)

Put broth and water in a large saucepan. Bring to a boil, add pasta, reduce heat and cover. Cook until tender, about ten minutes. Add beans and spinach. Heat through.

Per Serving:
Calories: 157 **Fat:** 1g **Carbohydrate:** 30g
Protein: 7g   **Sodium:** 550mg

SODIUM ALERT!
If you are on a sodium-restricted diet, then substitute, for example, Health Valley "no salt added" chicken broth and use, for example, Eden "very low sodium" canned navy beans.

Split Pea Soup
Floating Casserole III

6 servings

This recipe uses dried split peas. Unlike most other dried beans, they do not need to be soaked in advance. They should, however, be checked for the presence of small pebbles.

This is a good, thick soup. It will thicken as it cools, giving it a kind of magical quality. Since you'll have to add water each time you heat the soup, it will replenish itself.

1 16-ounce package dried split peas
2 1/2 quarts water
2 carrots, peeled and sliced, about 1 cup
1 large onion, coarsely chopped
1 large stalk celery, coarsely chopped, about 1/2 cup
1 teaspoon salt
1/2 teaspoon dried oregano

Put everything in a large pot. Bring to a boil, then cover and simmer gently until thick, about 1 1/2 hours.

Per Serving:
Calories: 160   **Fat:** 0g **Carbohydrate:** 30g
Protein: 10g   **Sodium:** 427mg

SODIUM ALERT!

If you are on a sodium-restricted diet, use your favorite salt substitute.

Fat-free Gravy
Makes 2 Cups (8 Servings)

You don't have to give up gravy! Fat is a significant part of most gravy recipes, but not this one.

1 13 3/4-ounce can defatted chicken broth (College Inn Lower Salt. Chill can for easy removal of fat.)

2 tablespoons cornstarch

1/4 cup water

1 teaspoon dried herbs, such as thyme or marjoram

Freshly ground pepper

1/4 teaspoon Kitchen Bouquet (for color)

Tabasco sauce (optional)

Bring the broth to a boil in a small saucepan. Meanwhile, stir the cornstarch into the water and mix well until dissolved. Using a wire whisk, add slowly to boiling broth, which will quickly thicken. Simmer a bit longer, just until gravy is clear and bubbly. Stir in herbs and pepper. Add Kitchen Bouquet. For gravy with a "bite," add a few drops of Tabasco to taste.

Per Serving:
Calories: 12 **Fat:** 0g **Carbohydrate:** 3g **Protein:** 0g **Sodium:** 137mg

Embarrassingly

Simple

Recipes

Our Favorite Oil and Vinegar Dressing
For 4 Servings of Salad

A typical salad dressing can be a part of low-fat living. If you generally go with low-fat and fat-free foods, you can use a delicious, "regular-fat" dressing on your salad. There's method in our madness, because when you eat salad, you are eating vegetables. (Just remember that this is a salad dressing, not a salad dousing.)

1/4 cup olive oil
1/8 cup balsamic or red wine vinegar
1 teaspoon Dijon mustard
Freshly ground pepper to taste

Combine all ingredients in a small jar. Shake well.

Per Serving:
Calories: 126 **Fat:** 14g **Carbohydrate:** 0g **Protein:** 0g **Sodium:** 17mg

Mandarin Orange and Red Onion

(the surprise combination)

4 Servings

This makes a nice change from salad, a pleasantly refreshing and color-ful side dish. And it needs no oil-based dressing.

2 11-ounce cans mandarin orange slices in light syrup
1/4 medium red onion, chopped
2 tablespoons red wine vinegar

Drain orange slices, but not too thoroughly. Toss with red onion and red wine vinegar.

Per Serving:
Calories: 48 **Fat:** 0g **Carbohydrate:** 11g **Protein:** 1g **Sodium:** 7mg

Embarrassingly

Simple

Recipes

Sun-dried Tomato Paste

Makes about 3/4 cup

Spread on fat-free crackers, this makes a delicious hors d'oeuvre. It's also great on chicken (see recipe for Chicken with Sun-Dried Tomato Paste, page 138).

1 8-ounce jar sun-dried tomatoes marinated in olive oil, very well drained
1 scallion, coarsely chopped
Freshly ground pepper

Put the sun-dried tomatoes and scallion in food processor bowl. Add a generous dose of pepper. Process until smooth.

Per Tablespoon:
Calories: 44 **Fat:** 3g **Carbohydrate:** 4g **Protein:** 1g **Sodium:** 6mg

A note on sun-dried tomatoes: Not only do they come marinated in oil, but also dried, in little cellophane packages. If you choose the dried ones (for salads and other dishes), don't try using them as is! They'll be harder to chew than tomato-flavored cardboard, and will taste like it, too. To soften: put tomatoes in a microwave container with enough water to cover them. Then "nuke" them, as the kids say, for 3 minutes. If you prefer (or have no microwave), put tomatoes in a small saucepan and cover with water. Bring to a boil, reduce heat, and simmer for about 5 minutes, or until tomatoes are very soft.

Yogurt-Mustard Sauce
Makes 1/2 cup

Embarrassingly

Simple

Recipes

This "sauce" makes a good dip for fresh vegetables, a tasty salad dressing, a fine marinade, and a wonderful accompaniment for fish (poached salmon, for example), cold or hot.

1/2 cup nonfat plain yogurt
1 teaspoon Dijon mustard
1 1/2 teaspoons fresh dill, chopped (optional. If you do use fresh dill, use only the thin, needle-like part, not the stems.)

Blend and taste. If you prefer more or less mustard, adjust proportions accordingly.

Per Tablespoon:
Calories: 16 **Fat:** 0g **Carbohydrate:** 2g **Protein:** 2g **Sodium:** 39mg

Embarrassingly

Simple

Recipes

Desserts

T here is life beyond a piece of fruit at dessert time, even on a low-fat diet.

French Toast with a Difference
4 Servings

Looks like breakfast, tastes like breakfast, but why not have it for dessert some cold winter night?

> **1/4 cup egg substitute, such as egg beaters**
> **1/2 cup skim milk**
> **1/2 teaspoon cinnamon**
> **1/4 teaspoon vanilla**
> **4 slices of your favorite bread**
> **All-fruit topping (can be found in the supermarket with the jams and jellies)**

Beat the egg substitute with the milk and cinnamon and vanilla. Soak bread, turning once, and cook in a nonstick skillet until brown. Heat the all-fruit topping over low heat and serve with the french toast.

Per Serving:
Calories: 152   **Fat:** 0g   **Carbohydrate:** 31g   **Protein:** 7g   **Sodium:** 209mg

Embarrassingly

Simple

Recipes

Egg White Omelet

A fast, delicious, treat

Makes one omelet

Like French Toast with a Difference, this is a breakfast dish that also makes a wonderful dessert. Keep in mind that it's egg yolks you are trying to avoid, since that's where the fat is. That leaves, by certain calculations, the whites. (Remember when you made hollandaise sauce and then tried to figure out what to do with the whites? Now you can use the whites and try to figure out what to do with the yolks.)

3 egg whites
2 teaspoons all-fruit jam

Beat egg whites with fork until very fluffy. Spray a small, nonstick skillet lightly with oil, heat, and add egg white mixture. Cook in the hot skillet for 1 minute, turn carefully, and cook other side for 15 to 30 seconds. Top with all-fruit jam.

Per Omelet:
Calories: 84   **Fat:** 0g   **Carbohydrate:** 11g   **Protein:** 10g   **Sodium:** 150mg

A Great Raspberry Sauce
Makes 1 cup (8 servings)

1 10-ounce package frozen raspberries in light syrup, thawed
1 tablespoon lemon juice
1 tablespoon orange liqueur (optional)

Put raspberries in food processor to purée. Strain to remove seeds if you're feeling ambitious. Add lemon juice; add orange liqueur if desired.

Per Serving:
Calories: 24 **Fat:** 0g **Carbohydrate:** 6g **Protein:** 0g **Sodium:** 0mg

Embarrassingly

Simple

Recipes

Pretty Apple Dessert with Three Options
4 Servings

This is a "three in one" recipe. For company, you might want to offer all three versions.

> **4 large hard, crunchy apples (Winesap, for example)**
> **1/4 cup all-fruit apricot preserves**
>   *OR*
> **1/4 teaspoon ground cinnamon mixed with 1 1/2 teaspoons sugar**
>   *OR*
> **1/2 cup A Great Raspberry Sauce (see previous recipe)**

Peel and slice apples. Arrange in single layer on nonstick baking sheet. Broil (not too near heat) until golden, about 15 minutes. If you will be using the preserves, melt over low heat while apples are cooking.

Arrange browned apple slices in a pie pan. Pour preserves over them OR sprinkle with the cinnamon-sugar mixture OR top with raspberry sauce. Serve warm.

Per Serving:
Calories: 128 **Fat:** 0g **Carbohydrate:** 32g **Protein:** 0g **Sodium:** 9mg

Fresh Berries with Frozen Yogurt and Raspberry Sauce
4 Servings

1 pint fresh berries, washed
1/2 cup A Great Raspberry Sauce (see recipe, page 181)
1 pint vanilla nonfat frozen yogurt
4 sprigs fresh mint (if available)

Using four pretty dishes (dishes can make all the difference), divide berries evenly, put a small scoopful of yogurt on top of berries in each dish, pour raspberry sauce over that, and garnish with mint.

Per Serving:
Calories: 144 **Fat:** 0g **Carbohydrate:** 33g **Protein:** 3g **Sodium:** 67mg

Embarrassingly

Simple

Recipes

Berries with NONFROZEN Yogurt
4 Servings

1 pint fresh berries, washed
**1 8-ounce container nonfat yogurt (not frozen yogurt) in any
fruit flavor you prefer**

Using four dishes, divide berries evenly and top with yogurt. You can
either match (blueberry yogurt on blueberries, strawberry yogurt on
strawberries) or mix (blueberry yogurt on strawberries, for instance).

Per Serving:
Calories: 79 **Fat:** 0g **Carbohydrate:** 18g **Protein:** 2g **Sodium:** 28mg

Really Nice Custard Dessert
4 Servings

1/4 cup sugar
2 cups skim milk
3/4 cup egg substitute, such as egg beaters
1 teaspoon vanilla
1/2 cup fresh berries (optional)

Preheat oven to 350°F.

Rinse a medium saucepan with cold water. (This will keep milk from sticking and make the pot easier to clean.) Combine milk and sugar, then heat almost to boiling, stirring to dissolve the sugar and to make sure you don't scorch the mixture. Remove from heat and gently mix in the egg substitute and the vanilla. Pour into four individual custard cups (oven-proof).

Set in a pan of hot water (or else you'll make four dried-out little cakes instead of custard), and bake for one hour. The custard will seem shivery when it comes out, but it solidifies as it cools. Chill. Top with fresh berries if you wish.

Per Serving:
Calories: 130 **Fat:** 2g **Carbohydrate:** 18g **Protein:** 10g **Sodium:** 146mg

Embarrassingly

Simple

Recipes

Pumpkin Pie-Less (no crust)
8 Servings

1 16-ounce can pumpkin, nothing added
1/2 cup egg substitute, such as egg beaters
1 teaspoon ground allspice
1/2 teaspoon ground ginger
1/4 teaspoon ground cloves
2/3 cup sugar
1 12-ounce can evaporated skim milk

Preheat oven to 400°F.

Combine all ingredients in a large bowl, blend well, and pour into 1-quart casserole dish, lightly sprayed with oil. Bake for 50 to 60 minutes. May be served warm or at room temperature.

Per Serving:
Calories: 137 **Fat:** 1g **Carbohydrate:** 26g **Protein:** 6g **Sodium:** 86mg

"Chocolate" Angel Food Cake

(Made from a mix, of course)

12 Servings

1 box Angel Food Cake mix
1/2 cup unsweetened cocoa powder

Follow package directions. Before pouring batter into tube pan, add the cocoa powder and blend in well. Continue to follow directions as given on the box.

Per Serving:
Calories: 152 **Fat:** 0g **Carbohydrate:** 33g **Protein:** 5g **Sodium:** 142mg

Embarrassingly

Simple

Recipes

Embarrassingly

Simple

Recipes

Vanilla Soufflé to Remember

6 Servings

This is the one NON-embarrassingly simple recipe, and has been included because it takes low-fat cooking to new heights. People think that soufflés are difficult to make, and that really isn't true.

When you look at the recipe analysis, you may be surprised to see that there is more fat per serving than we have been recommending, and indeed the recipe calls for 1 1/2 teaspoons rather than one teaspoon of added fat. Otherwise, it follows our rules, incorporating monounsaturated fat (canola oil) and fat-free dairy products (skim milk). In addition, by using an egg substitute such as egg beaters instead of eggs, a fair amount of fat is eliminated. So – this soufflé becomes a wonderful, special treat, a fine celebration of all your efforts to reduce the fat in your daily diet.

Let's try this together.

Prepare a 2-quart soufflé dish as follows:

Using spray oil, lightly coat the inside of the dish, bottom and sides. Put in a couple of tablespoons of sugar, rotate dish so sugar clings to oil on bottom and sides, and dump out excess.

Now for the soufflé:

> **3 tablespoons canola oil**
> **3 tablespoons flour**
> **1 cup skim milk**
> **1/3 cup sugar**
> **1 cup egg substitute, such as egg beaters**
> **2 teaspoons vanilla**
> **8 egg whites, at room temperature**
> **1 pint nonfat chocolate frozen yogurt, mostly melted**

Preheat oven to 350°F.

Put oil and flour in a saucepan. Using a wire whisk, mix together over moderate heat, stirring constantly. When mixture bubbles, add the milk and sugar. Continue to heat and stir. Lower heat slightly and add egg substitute. DO NOT STOP STIRRING, or you will wind up with something that is so clotted you won't be able to blend it with the egg whites in the next step. Continue to stir until mixture is thickened and smooth. Remove from heat and stir in vanilla. Set aside.

Using a large bowl, beat egg whites until stiff but not dry. With an electric mixer this will take several minutes. When you run a rubber spatula through the middle, it should leave a trough. (Another test is that it forms stiff peaks when you pull the spatula up, not little points that sort of fall over.) Pour in the cooled egg substitute mixture and, using that same rubber spatula, fold gently into the whites, so that the air will stay in the egg whites and allow the soufflé to rise impressively. (If you've never folded anything but laundry: With your palm down, keeping the spatula flat against the bowl, pull it along under the mixture and sort of roll it over the top, turning your palm up as you do so. Turn the bowl a bit and repeat. Keep doing this until the yellow egg substitute mixture has combined with the egg whites and the whole thing is a uniform pale yellow. Be gentle as you perform this operation. What you are trying to do is KEEP THE AIR IN THE EGG WHITES.)

Pour into the prepared soufflé dish and bake for about 30 minutes, or until the top is golden brown and dry. (Do not peek during cooking, unless you have one of those ovens with a little window and a light inside.) This is the time for everyone to come and admire, because once you start scooping out the portions with a large serving spoon, the soufflé will begin to collapse. That's fine, though. It will still taste wonderful. Serve with 1/4 cup of the mostly melted frozen yogurt on the side of each plate.

Per Serving:
Calories: 236 **Fat:** 8g **Carbohydrate:** 29g **Protein:** 12g **Sodium:** 194mg

Inspiration

To Keep You
On The Low-Fat Track

For Those Moments When You Wonder
How in the World You Got Yourself into This

Remember:

☞ When it comes to low-fat living, you know that any step, no matter how small, is a step in the right direction.

☞ You are feeling better generally.

☞ You look better, and you may even be shedding some unwanted pounds.

☞ You have taken control of your health in a major way, maybe even extending your life.

☞ You are doing something wonderful for your family – and for yourself.

For Further Information

Free! Free! Free! An array of publications to help you adapt to low-fat living, including well-designed, colorful pamphlets for the younger generation. Simply send your request(s), along with your name and address, to:

National Heart, Blood and Lung Institute
Information Center
P.O. Box 30105
Bethesda, Maryland 20824-0105

The publications:

"So You Have High Blood Cholesterol"
"Step by Step: Eating to Lower Your High Blood Cholesterol"

For seven- to ten-year-olds:
"Eating with Your Heart in Mind"

For eleven- to fourteen-year-olds:
"Heart Health . . . Your Choice"

For fifteen- to eighteen-year-olds:
"Healthy Heart Habits"

A Parent's Guide:
"Cholesterol in Children: Healthy Eating is a Family Affair"

For more information about the Food Guide Pyramid, as well as a colorful picture of it, write for the Pyramid pamphlet. Mail your request with your name and address, together with a one-dollar check made out to the "Superintendent of Documents," to:

Consumer Information Service
Department 159Z
United States Department of Agriculture
Pueblo, Colorado 81009

Here is a very short list of cookbooks that contain some wonderful, low-fat recipes. You may have to make slight revisions to stay with the four points you now know by heart:

❶ Think 3-ounce serving sizes of Extra Lean meat, fish, or chicken.

❷ Use low-fat or fat-free dairy products.

❸ Use monounsaturated fats, the "fats of choice"– olive and canola oils.

❹ Try to keep recipes near 1 teaspoon added fat per serving.

Jane Brody's Good Food Book, Jane Brody (New York: Bantam Books), 1987.

Jane Brody's Good Food Gourmet, Jane Brody (New York: W.W. Norton & Company), 1990.

Eat Smart for a Healthy Heart Cookbook, revised edition, Denton A. Cooley, M.D. and Carolyn E. Moore, Ph.D., R.D. (Hauppauge, NY: Barron's Educational Series), 1992.

The American Heart Association Low-Fat, Low-Cholesterol Cookbook, Scott Grundy and Mary Winston, editors (New York: Random House), 1991.

Eat More, Weigh Less, Dean Ornish, M.D. (NY: HarperCollins), 1993.

Other good resources:

"Cooking Light: The Magazine of Food and Fitness," published bimonthly by Southern Living, Inc.
Call (800) 336-0125 for subscription information.

"Nutrition Action Healthletter," published monthly by the Center for Science in the Public Interest
1875 Connecticut Avenue, N.W.
Suite 300
Washington, DC 20009-5728
Or call (202) 332-9110 for subscription information.

Endnotes

Particular mention must be made of the **FEDERAL REGISTER, Volume 58, No. 3, Wednesday, January 6, 1993**, which contains Food and Drug Administration (FDA) regulations set forth in the Nutrition Labeling and Education Act. The Food Safety and Inspection Service (FSIS), responsible for labeling certain meat and poultry products, parallel the FDA regulations "to the extent possible."

1. Several important studies in the last fifteen years have identified a fatty substance in the blood that is associated with heart disease, and is called – you guessed it – cholesterol. However, in and of itself it is not a villain, but is an integral part of animal cell structure and a major component of brain tissue. In other words, without cholesterol we would be cell-less and brain-less. Cholesterol is so important that the liver produces what the body needs.

2. Jane Brody, *Jane Brody's New York Times Guide to Personal Health* (New York: Times Books), 1982, p. 24.

3. Overeating fat can make a person fatter than can overeating starches.
    Y. Schutz, J.P. Flatt, E. Jequier, "Failure of Dietary Fat Intake to Promote Fat Oxidation: A Factor Favoring the Development of Obesity," *American Journal of Clinical Nutrition*, 50:307-14, 1989.
    L. Shepperd, A.R. Kristal, L.H. Kushi, "Weight Loss in Women Participating in a Randomized Trial of Low Fat Diets," *American Journal of Clinical Nutrition*, 54:821-8, 1991.

4. How do you know if you're eating a lot of sugar? Sugars can be

found in various disguises, so check the Ingredient List for any of these obvious sugars – corn syrup, molasses, honey, brown sugar – as well as these less obvious ones: glucose, sucrose, fructose, levulose, maltose, whey, mannitol, and sorbitol.

There are no studies that show that sugar causes heart disease (just cavities). But while it can't hurt, it doesn't help. Sugar contains no vitamins, minerals, or fiber, and by taking in energy in the form of sugar, you tend not to eat foods that are good for you: fruits, vegetables, and starches.

5. Nutrition Labeling and Education Act of 1990. *Federal Register*, volume 58, number 3, January 6, 1993, p. 654.

6. "Beans, Beans, the musical fruit,
   The more you eat, the more you toot.
   The more you toot, the better you feel,
   So eat baked beans at every meal."

7. Rinsing canned beans before using them, or soaking dried beans and discarding that water before cooking them in fresh water, will help decrease flatulence.

8. Starchy beans, as well as oats and barley, contain soluble fiber, which lowers serum cholesterol levels.
   S.R. Glore, Ph.D., R.D.; D. Van Treeck, M.S., R.D.; A.W. Knehaus, Ph.D., et al., "Soluble Fiber and Serum Lipids: A Literature Review," *Journal of the American Dietetic Association*, 94: 425–36, 1994.

9. Current research shows that fruits and vegetables contain thousands of compounds, many of which are only now beginning to be studied. While there is still a pleasant mystery to the whole thing, we do know that fruits and vegetables pack a health wallop, and that it is far better to eat these foods than it is to take vitamin and mineral supplements.

10. Yes, believe it or not, in a nationwide survey conducted from 1976 to 1980, 45 percent of those contacted had consumed no fruit or fruit juice that day.

    B.H. Patterson, G. Block, W.F. Rosenberger, et al., "Fruit and Vegetables in the American Diet: Data from the National Health and Nutrition Examination Survey," *American Journal of Public Health*, 80:1443-9, 1990.

11. It doesn't take much protein to make new cells, et cetera, and most people eat more than they need. Unless you have a specific medical reason, you do not need to worry about eating too little protein. (If you are concerned that you have special protein needs, seek professional advice.) As long as you eat a wide variety of starches and vegetables, you'll be getting plenty of protein, and you'll be eating less fat.

12. V. Fonnebo, "Mortality in Norwegian Seventh-Day Adventists 1962-1986," *Journal of Clinical Epidemiology*, 45(2):157-67, 1992.

    M. Kestin and I.L. Rouse, "Cardiovascular Disease Risk Factors in Free-Living Men: Comparison of Two Prudent Diets, One Based on Lactoovovegetarianism and the other allowing Lean Meat," *American Journal of Clinical Nutrition*, 50(2):280-87, 1989.

13. Just in case your meat department doesn't have readily available information, or if the "meat in question" doesn't say "Extra Lean" or "Lean," you can fall back on the old method of consulting a list of cuts of meat that qualify.

    (Note that these are "extra lean" only if you eat no more than three ounces. The more you eat, the more fat you'll get.)

"EXTRA LEAN" CUTS OF MEAT
No more than 5g of fat (2g saturated) in 3 ounces

Beef	Game	Pork	Poultry (skinless)
Eye round tenderloin	Venison	Cured ham, butt end	Chicken breast turkey breast

"LEAN" CUTS OF MEAT
No more than 10g of fat (4g saturated) in 3 ounces

Beef	Pork	Poultry (skinless)
Flank steak (fat trimmed), top round, bottom round, rump	Canned ham (shank end), fresh lean ham	Dark meat of turkey and chicken (*Except chicken wings! Very high in fat*)

14. D. Kromhout, E.B. Bosschieter, C. Coulander, "The Inverse Relation Between Fish Consumption and 20-year Mortality From Coronary Heart Disease," New England Journal of Medicine, 312:1205-09, 1985.

15. Even though shellfish is very, very low in fat, it does not qualify as "extra lean" or "lean" because it contains too much cholesterol to qualify. But don't be fooled by the name. The "cholesterol" in shellfish seems to be different, maybe even beneficial.

    M.T. Childs, C.S. Dorsett, A. Failor, et al., "Effect of Shellfish Consumption on Cholesterol Absorption in Normolipidemic Men," *Metabolism: Clinical and Experimental*, 36(1):31-35, 1987.

16. If you decide to give up high-fat cheese, don't throw out the baby with the bath water. You still need a source of calcium, which you can get from low-fat and fat-free dairy products. Without them, you probably need calcium supplements. Check with a doctor or registered dietitian.

17. Consumption of partially hydrogenated vegetable oils (it's that *trans* fat) may contribute to coronary heart disease.

    W. Willett, M. Stampfer, J. Mason, et al., "Intake of *Trans* Fatty Acids and Risk of Coronary Heart Disease Among Women," *Lancet*, 341:581-85, 1993.

    For a review of the literature:

    W. Willet, M.D., D.P.H., and A. Ascherio, M.D., D.P.H., "*Trans*

Fatty Acids: Are the Effects Only Marginal?" *American Journal of Public Health*, 84:722-24, 1994.

18. This means that there is no protein and no carbohydrate in margarine. All the calories come from fat. Even if it is a reduced-calorie version, there are simply fewer calories, but they all come from fat.

19. While this appears to be a trend in epidemiological studies, it is possible that there are other factors responsible for the low rate of heart disease in Mediterranean countries.

20. Like olive oil, canola oil is predominately monounsaturated. And it has even less saturated fat.

21. One teaspoon of fat is equal to:

 1/6 avocado
 5 large olives
 10 small olives
 6 almonds
 3 jumbo cashews
 10 peanuts (large)
 2 teaspoons peanut butter
 2 whole pecans
 18 pistachios

22. Here's how we've arrived at those 65 grams:

 1 teaspoon of fat = 5 grams
 13 teaspoons of fat = 65 grams
 That is, 13 x 5 = 65

Incidentally:

 1 gram of fat = 9 calories
 65 grams of fat = 585 calories
 (That is, 65 x 9 = 585)

23. When you saw that little number, you thought we were going to list the "many, many texts available on the subject," didn't you? Instead, we'll make one suggestion. Like the other texts, this comes complete with charts that will help you determine "your daily fat-grams budget," as this book calls it. Joseph Piscatella, *Controlling Your Fat Tooth* (New York: Workman Publishing), 1991.

24. For more information about introducing new foods to children, see: Ellyn Satter, *How to Get Your Kid to Eat . . . But Not Too Much* (Palo Alto, CA: Bull Publishing Co.), 1987.

25. If you are concerned about sodium, look for foods that say:
"Low sodium" (140mg or less per serving)
"Very low sodium" (35mg or less per serving)
"Sodium-free" (less than 5mg per serving)

26. Dorothea Van Gundy Jones, *The Soybean Cookbook* (New York: Arco Publishing Co., Inc.), 1974, p. 5.

27. Terms on labels that are useful in helping you eat less fat:

"Fat Free"– less than 0.5g total fat per serving.

"Low Fat"– 3g or less total fat per serving. ("Low Fat" may not be a bargain if their serving size is only two crackers. Again, check your OPSS.)

"Extra Lean"– no more than 5 grams of total fat, 2 grams of saturated fat, in a 3-ounce serving.

"Lean"– no more than 10 grams of total fat, 4 grams of saturated fat, in a 3-ounce serving.

NOT SO FAST! CHECK LABELS FURTHER BEFORE ASSUMING LOW TOTAL FAT.

"Low Saturated Fat"– 1g or less saturated fat per serving. *Does not necessarily mean the product is low in total fat.*

"Less Fat," "Reduced Fat"– 25 percent less total fat than the original version. (It may be worth taking a look at the original version, which might be so high in fat that a 25 percent reduction still leaves an awful lot in there.)

"Light"– contains 1/3 the calories or 1/2 the fat of the original version of the food. Technically a product can be called "light" by reducing calories only, which still leaves the product with the original amount of fat. Also, you can have a "light" product with 50 percent fat. As an example, margarine is 100 percent fat and can be called "light" if its fat content is reduced by 50 percent (the other 50 percent is air). It's still all fat, though.

"Low Cholesterol"– less than 20mg per serving, and less than 2g saturated fat per serving. You could still be eating a high-fat product. *"Low cholesterol" does not mean low fat.*

28. Wayne Gisslen, *Professional Cooking* (New York: John Wiley and Sons), 1983, p. 318.

29. There is inconsistency in claims made on and off food packages since they are regulated by different government agencies. While the FDA regulates claims on the food labels themselves, the Federal Trade Commission (FTC) regulates food advertisements in the media. Because the FTC apparently has better things to do than check out misleading nutrition claims, they are found all too often in advertisements that appear in print and on television.

30. "Single ingredient raw foods" include fresh produce, raw fish, meat, and poultry. Labeling on these foods is strictly voluntary, but who needs labels on fresh fruits and vegetables anyway? Meat and poultry are a different story altogether. We need specific information for

each cut of meat. Nutrition information is probably somewhere in the store, but it may be hard to get. Too bad. We need it.

31. Here is some general comparative information about the fat content of various lunch meats, cheeses, and mayonnaise-based salads.

   Different brands of lunch meat contain slightly different amounts of fat, but this will give you a good idea of what you're dealing with. Remember, you are looking for Extra Lean and Lean meats.

Product	Serving size	Amount of fat
Turkey breast	two slices (two ounces)	2.0g
Ham (extra lean)	"	2.8g
Turkey salami	"	6.8g
Regular salami	"	10.0g
Bologna	"	6.5g

Pretty thin sandwich you have there. Are you sure you eat only two slices? Think OPSS (Own Personal Serving Size).

   Cheeses are another question altogether. We can tell you how much fat is in an ounce of a given cheese, but then again, you think of eating a *piece* of cheese, not an ounce of cheese, so you're probably wondering what that one ounce looks like. Was it cut from a brick of cheese? A wedge? Is it prepackaged, with those little pieces of paper in between the slices? Is it sliced at the deli counter, so that a piece of Swiss is approximately the size of a notepad? And how about grated cheese? The next time you're at the supermarket, treat yourself to an ounce of a number of different shaped cheeses, and you'll begin to get used to what an ounce looks like.

Product	Serving size	Amount of fat
Mozzarella	one ounce	7g
Parmesan	"	7g
Swiss	"	8g
American	"	9g
Cheddar	"	9g

As you can see, cheese is high in fat, so if you are determined to eat a lot of it, you might want to examine high-tech cheeses, on which the terms "fat free" or "low fat" will surely appear. Manufacturers have managed to take all or some of the fat out of them, but you are likely to find that the taste has also been taken out, and when you try to heat the cheese, you are left with something that looks as if it should be played with rather than eaten.

Mayonnaise-based products: Note that one ounce of these salads is only about 1/8 cup. Chances are that you eat more than that, probably at least half a cup, which contains 4 times the fat that is listed here. That is, an average serving of one of these salads would contain about 16 grams of fat.

Product	Serving size	Amount of fat
Chicken salad	one ounce	4.0g
Ham salad	"	4.5g
Potato salad	"	3.0g
Macaroni salad	"	4.0g

Meat information is based on J. Pope-Cordle and M. Katahn, *The Low-Fat Supermarket Shopper's Guide* (New York: W.W. Norton and Company, New York), 1993, and J. Pennington, *Bowes and Church's Food Values of Portions Commonly Used*, 16th ed. (Philadelphia, PA: J.B. Lippincott Company), 1994.

Cheese information is based on *Bowes and Church's Food Values of Portions Commonly Used*, above.

Salad information is based on J. Pope-Cordle and M. Katahn, *The T-Factor Fat Gram Counter* (New York: W.W. Norton and Company), 1991, and *Bowes and Church's Food Values of Portions Commonly Used*, above.

32. Angiographic studies ("up close and personal" looks inside the arteries) show that a low-fat diet decreases the amount of plaque ("gunk") in the arteries of the heart. The lower the total fat in the diet, the greater the improvement.

In the STARS study, a 27 percent-fat diet was followed. Plaque decreased in 38 percent of the participants.

In the Lifestyle Heart Study, conducted by Dean Ornish, participants followed a 10 percent-fat diet; arterial plaque decreased in 82 percent of the individuals studied.

The Ornish study included other significant lifestyle changes as well, such as daily meditation, three hours of exercise per week, and weekly group therapy sessions. Following such a regimen was difficult but rewarding for participants and those who cared about them.

You might want to take a look at *Dr. Dean Ornish's Program for Reversing Heart Disease* (NY: Random House), 1990.

33. "How can I find out my precise calorie needs?" we hear you say. For a true measure, you can go to the pulmonary-rehabilitation department at any major hospital and be hooked up to a piece of high-tech equipment. Or you can go to a registered dietitian for a "calculated energy needs" assessment.

34. Where does that 65 grams of fat come from? If you consume 2,000 calories a day, and you figure that 30 percent of those calories can come from fat, that means 600 calories a day can come from fat.

Now, if you look at the last line of the food label, you'll see that there are 9 calories in a gram of fat. Do the calculation (divide 600 calories by 9 grams of fat per calorie), and you'll find this is equivalent to approximately 65 grams of fat.

Aren't you glad you read this note?

35. For those interested in the math behind this easy to use screening device, otherwise known as 5% Daily Value:

The Nutrition Labeling and Education Act has given specific guidelines for "low" Total Fat, Saturated Fat, Cholesterol, and Sodium. The figures are given in metric measurements, which is to say grams and milligrams.

By taking the value for "low" and dividing by the Daily Value, we

Endnotes

get 5%. Take Total Fat for example:

$$\frac{3 \text{ grams}}{65 \text{ grams}} = 5\%$$

You can do the same math for Saturated Fat, Cholesterol, and Sodium. The result will be the same – or something close to it.

36. Unfortunately, the "sugars" listing is confusing, because it includes sugars that occur naturally as well as those that have been added. Therefore milk and fruits look as if they are high in sugars when that's really not an issue at all (*Federal Register*, pp. 2097-2098).

37. "Based on current scientific evidence . . . protein intake is not a public health concern for adults . . . ." *Food Labeling Questions and Answers*, Office of Food Labeling, Food and Drug Administration, August 1993, p. 3.

38. The "Embarrassingly Simple Recipes" stay within government guidelines for heart-healthy foods (*Federal Register*, pp. 2494-95):

	Single Food	Main Dish
Total Fat (g)	13	19.5
Saturated Fat (g)	4	6
Cholesterol (mg)	60	90
Sodium (mg)	480	720

Exceptions are shrimp (Shrimp with Tomatoes) and pink salmon (Crunchy Tuna Salad made with salmon); both are higher in cholesterol than suggested in the guidelines. We have included them because other aspects of all seafood and fish make them fine additions to a heart-healthy diet.

39. Sodium alerts offer suggestions for keeping sodium levels under 140 mg per serving of a single food and 500 mg per main dish.

Index